A Brief History of Āyurveda

A Brief History of Āyurveda

M.R. RAGHAVA VARIER

OXFORD
UNIVERSITY PRESS

OXFORD
UNIVERSITY PRESS

Oxford University Press is a department of the University of Oxford. It furthers the University's objective of excellence in research, scholarship, and education by publishing worldwide. Oxford is a registered trademark of Oxford University Press in the UK and in certain other countries.

Published in India by
Oxford University Press
22 Workspace, 2nd Floor, 1/22 Asaf Ali Road, New Delhi 110002, India

First Edition published in 2020

ISBN-13 (print edition): 978-0-19-012108-2
ISBN-10 (print edition): 0-19-012108-4

ISBN-13 (eBook): 978-0-19-099210-1
ISBN-10 (eBook): 0-19-099210-7

Typeset in ScalaPro 10/12.4
by Tranistics Data Technologies, Kolkata 700 091
Printed in India by Rakmo Press, New Delhi 110 020

Contents

List of Figures and Tables vii
Preface ix
Acknowledgements xi
Scheme of Transliteration xiii
Introduction: Historiography of Āyurveda xv

1. Early Historic Phase 1
2. Towards Scientific Foundations of Healing: Buddhist Heterodox Tradition 22
3. The Age of the Samhitas 40
4. *Suśrutasamhita* 66
5. Samhitas of Bhēḷa, Haritha, and Kasyapa, and Other Samhitas 85
6. Ancient Indian Medical Education 95
7. Regional Developments 101
8. Experiment with Modernity: The Decline and Reawakening of Āyurveda 117

Concluding Observations 123
Appendix: Auxiliary Branches of Knowledge: Treatment for Plants and Animals 130
Selected Glossary 159
Selected Readings 162
Index 165
About the Author 173

Figures and Tables

Figures

2.1 Medicine Box 24
2.2 Girnar Edict II 37

4.1 Surgical Tools 69

7.1 Thirumukkutal Inscription: Medicines Stored in the Hospital Attached to the Temple 107

Tables

3.1 The Lineage of *Ācārya*s and Their Preceptors 43

7.1 Remuneration Given to Staff Members of the Medical Institution 110

Preface

Following a general trend, Āyurveda is often officially described and commonly known even among its practitioners as 'alternative medicine', whereas the available sources clearly show that it was the mainstream healthcare programme in the subcontinent for roughly more than two-and-a-half millennia in the past. This is perhaps the result of an inherent indifference to the historical background of developments in the indigenous science of medicine and healthcare. Medicine and its practice do not exist in a vacuum, nor do they flourish without economic and social necessities. There is no dearth of literature on the history of Āyurveda but most of the available works are in the form of descriptive accounts of or discussions on the content of the classics, their commentaries, and so on. Generally speaking, these volumes seldom make any attempt to place the developments that occur from time to time in the system of Āyurveda in their historical context. This is perhaps due to the approaches, which are, as a rule, myopic when it comes to the archaeological and epigraphic sources that shed light on many dimly lit areas of the topic. Access to a proper intellectual apparatus and ideational acumen with an appropriate theoretical frame is essential for a meaningful explanation of medicine and its practice in India, with special reference to their historical context. The present volume is a humble attempt at viewing the stages of development of Āyurveda, which was the mainstream indigenous medicine, and its practice, and at placing them in their historical context.

I have paid due attention, wherever necessary, to establishing linkages between the processes of history and social formation on the one side and the developments in the knowledge and practice of the science of Āyurveda on the other. This was possible thanks to the supporting evidences from a large number of medieval epigraphic documents and structural remains as well as archaeological artefacts from stratified layers. This is perhaps the prime relevance of a text such as this in the midst of a vast amount of literature produced by learned scholars and physicians in the past.

Any discussion of the knowledge of Āyurveda would be incomplete without a consideration of some allied branches of knowledge, such as the treatments for animals and plants. Hence, I have included a section on the relevant topics of Aśvāyurveda, treatment for horses; Hastyāyurveda, treatment for elephants; and Vṛkṣāyurveda, treatment for plants; and so forth, in the present text.

This volume is aimed at providing useful knowledge of the science of Āyurveda and its stages of development over the course of its existence for more than three millennia without serious breaks. It is my hope that this will help readers view the major achievements of this indigenous branch of medicine in their true sense, devoid of attempts at various levels on the part of the authorities to describe it and situate it as 'alternative medicine'.

M.R. Raghava Varier
31 December 2019

Acknowledgements

I was introduced to the subject of Āyurveda when I was invited to prepare a brief history of the Arya Vaidya Sala, Kottakkal, Kerala, on the occasion of the centenary celebrations of the institute in 2002. During the preparation of that work, I benefitted a lot from discussions with stalwarts such as Dr K. Rajagopal and Dr P.K. Warrier. Recently, I had to engage myself more seriously with the subject when I took up the role of chief editor in the Department of Publication, Arya Vaidya Sala. I have received immense help and assistance from several of my colleagues, including Dr K.V. Rajagopal and Dr Sunitha in the course of writing this book. I am extremely thankful to these institutions, scholars, and physicians for their help and support in collecting and organizing the materials.

Access to a variety of sources of information such as excavated materials, structural remains, and inscriptions in addition to literary texts is vital for such an enquiry. The office of the director of epigraphy, Archaeological Survey of India, Mysore, provided the most valued help by allowing me to examine the estampages of a large number of unpublished temple inscriptions preserved in their office. I am indebted to this institute for all its generous help. Professor Y. Subbarayalu provided me with the texts of several epigraphic records published in official publications, including the relevant volumes of South Indian inscriptions. I am thankful to Professor Subbarayalu for his indispensible support. During my research for the present study, I had the benefit of holding discussions with several physicians and scholars. My thanks are due to these scholars for their invaluable help, without which I would not have been able to complete this book.

Professor M.V. Narayanan of the Department of English, Calicut University, Kerala, took out time from his busy schedule to go through the draft version of this work and provide important feedback for enhancing the style and quality of the content of this work. Professor Kesavan Veluthat of the Department of History, Delhi University, also sat with me and went through some early versions of the present work. I take this opportunity to place on record my sincere gratitude to these friends for their invaluable help.

Scheme of Transliteration

Vowels

a ā i ī u ū e ai o ō

Consonants

ka kha ga gha ṅa
ca cha ja jha ña
ṭa ṭha ḍa ḍha ṇa
ta tha da dha na
pa pha ba bha ma
ya ra la va
śa ṣa sa ha

Dravidian Sounds

ḷa ḻa ṛa ṉa

Introduction

Historiography of Āyurveda

A quick survey of the historiography of Indian medicine would show that the subject has invited scholarly attention from at least the mid-nineteenth century onwards, when a large number of foreign scholars and native experts presented their views on various topics pertaining to the nature and evolution of the science of Āyurveda. A large corpus of literature has been produced on the subject. It is not our aim here to list them or to present a critique of the entire literature on the topic.

My present attempt is restricted to highlighting some major areas that were left dim in studies done in recent times due mainly to the nature of sources and equally to the perspective. It is also our aim to explain the new developments in terms of their historical context. At the same time, it is necessary to examine the points of view that exercised control over the writing and determined the tone of the studies. To cite an example, some scholars of the earlier part of the last century, such as H.T. Colebrook, who were preoccupied with the idea of a glorious Indian past, argued that the Hindus were teachers and not learners to establish that India owed nothing to foreign civilizations regarding the science of medicine. Some others, such as Stuart J. Pocock, went to the extent of saying that Pythagoras, the father of the art of healing in Greece, was originally an Indian whose name was Buddhaguru. Diaz Castillo was of the opinion that the medicinal culture of ancient Egypt was of Indian origin.[1] Contrary to this view was an incurable prejudice that suggested an implausible identification of Suśruta, the pioneering master of Indian surgical tradition who hailed from Kāśi, as Socrates, the Greek philosopher who was a native of Kos.[2] A perusal of the major works helps us identify certain trends that influenced the various perspectives of the historians dealing with almost the same source materials.[3] Mention may be made of an Orientalist section and a Nationalist section, both having subgroups that had their own views on specific issues and areas of the subject. Looking from a broad perspective, it may be observed that the Orientalists constructed a glorious image of the Indian past, while the Nationalists traced all knowledge systems to ancient Indian civilization. Serious works have doubtlessly been produced on the history of medicine in other cultures and other languages. Some of them may serve as a model for the new venture. The most prominent among them is the celebrated work of Joseph Needham, *Science and Civilization in China*. Works of Ralph Jackson, such as *Doctors and Diseases in the Roman Empire* (1988), and of Mirko D. Grmek, such as *Diseases in the Ancient Greek World* (1989), are also important contributions to the subject. A large number of scholars from different cultures and disciplines have since then attempted to trace the history of Āyurveda from various points of view.

The subject witnessed revived interest with the advent of the British Raj, towards the end of the eighteenth century CE. Occasional writings and casual references apart, systematic enquiries and the study of various aspects of Indian knowledge and wisdom were started with the establishment of the Asiatic Society of Bengal in 1784, thanks to the efforts of great scholars and Indologists such as Sir William Jones and H.H. Wilson. However, the interest of these pioneering scholars was confined, not without reason, mainly to the areas of literary and *Dharmaśāstra* texts. A casual examination of the corpus of these previous studies would show that while many of them brought out interesting details about the subject, they still suffered from

1 From Jean Filliozat, *The Classical Doctrines of Indian Medicine*, trans. Dev Raj Chanana (Delhi: Munshiram Manoharlal, 1964).

2 Johann Hermann Baas quoted in R. Niranjana, *Medicine in South India* (Chennai: Eswar Press, 2004), 52.

3 Narendra Bhatt, 'Indigenous Science of Healing and Healthcare', *Satabhisheka Smaranika* (Kottakal: Arya Vaidya Sala, 2005), 83–6.

inaccessibility to the required sources for a reasonable understanding of the subject.

Earlier scholars were biased, with different understandings and partisan world views. They presented their knowledge of the subject, quite naturally, solely on the basis of sources to which they had access. Thus, John Fleming wrote an essay about Indian herbs that could be used as medicine.[4] This was followed by another attempt with an interest in the materia medica of Indian medicine.[5] Preliminary observations on the state of early 'hindoo' medicine including surgery were published anonymously by H.H. Wilson in the *Oriental Magazine*, Calcutta, in 1823.[6] Surgeons of the East India Company were required officially to take note of any useful treatment carried out by Indian physicians. J.F. Royle was entrusted with the work of investigating the materia medica of India. He published his findings in 'An Essay in the Antiquity of Hindu Medicine' including an introductory lecture to the cause of materia medica and therapeutics delivered at King's College, London (1837). His source materials mainly consisted of collections from the bazaars and some native works on the subject. He concluded his study with the observation that there was some connection among the Indian, the Arabic, the Greek, and the Chinese traditions of medicine. T.A. Wise, another physician, examined the Hindu medical *sastra* by translating and comparing different manuscripts available to him. His interest was in establishing that India was a repository of medical knowledge and, in any case, also in refuting opinions to the contrary.[7] A balanced view on this issue was held at a later period by A.L. Basham who opined that 'the development of medicine also was probably stimulated by contact with Hellenic physicians and the resemblances between Indian and classical medicine suggest borrowing on both sides'. He added that:

[4] John Fleming, 'A Catalogue of Indian Medicinal Plants and Drugs, with Their Names in the Hindustani and Sanscrit Languages', *Asiatic Researches*, 1812, 11: 153–96. See also Deepak Kumar, 'Diseases and Medicine in India—A Historical Overview', paper presented at Proceedings of the Indian History Congress, New Delhi, 2001.

[5] Ainsle Whitelaw, *Materia Medica of Hindoostan* (Calcutta, 1813).

[6] H.H. Wilson, 'On the Native Practice in Cholera, with Remarks', *Oriental Magazine*, 1824, 2.

[7] T.A. Wise, *Commentary on the Hindu System of Medicine* (Calcutta: Messrs Thacker and Co., and Messrs Ostell, Lepage and Co., 1845).

> The basic conception of Indian medicine like that of ancient Europe was the humors wind, gall and mucus to which some added a fourth one blood. Despite their inaccurate knowledge of physiology which was by no means inferior to that of most ancient people, India evolved a developed empirical surgery. The caesarian section was known, bone setting reached a high degree of skill. Plastic surgery was developed far beyond anything known elsewhere at that time. Ancient Indian surgeons were experts at the repair of nose, ear and lips lost or injured in battle or by judicial mutilation. Indian surgery in this respect remained ahead of its European until the 18th century when the surgeons of the East India company were not ashamed to learn the art of rhinoplasty from the Indians.[8]

The administrative policy of the East India Company was, in the beginning, to provide support for the study and research of indigenous traditions of healing and healthcare, but this was reversed towards the first half of the nineteenth century. The history of Āyurveda was looked at from an Orientalist perspective by a set of scholars and they described the whole system as magico-religious and even superstitious. Evidently, these scholars had no access to the original sources of the Indian science of medicine. It is significant to note in this connection that the topic was well noticed and discussed by the traditional authorities themselves and a transition from the *daivavyapāśraya* (magico-religious) to the *yuktivyapāśraya* (empirical) finds expression in basic texts, such as the Samhitas. The earliest reference to this conceptual frame and a brief discussion on the issue is met with in the *Carakasamhita*, where the topic is presented with scientific rigour.[9] In 1833, the Grant Commission recommended that funds be granted for the teaching of Western medicine only. The commission also recorded that help and support for Indian medicine should be completely withdrawn. However, some French and German scholars strongly supported engagement with the study of Āyurveda. Generally speaking, the attention of Western scholarship during this period was mainly focused on the question of the interrelationship between Indian and Greek traditions of medicine. There was also a view that all the sciences originated in ancient Greece and that there

[8] A.L. Basham, *The Wonder That Was India* (Calcutta: Orient Longman, 1963), 499.

[9] *Carakasamhita*, ch. 1–58 and ch. 11–54. For further details see section on *Carakasamhita* in Chapter III.

was no science other than Greek science. Needless to say, this was an excessive claim influenced by an Orientalist view of Western scholarship. Julius Jolly, a German scholar, published a work in German titled *Medicine* (1901). This study includes a survey of the history of Indian medicine based on detailed critical study of a wide range of medical works from the Vedas to the Āyurvedic texts of the nineteenth century, which were chronologically arranged and dated. Apart from this, he mentioned some Buddhist texts, the Bower manuscript, medical glossaries, and works on veterinary sciences. This scholar, it is interesting to note, warned against the overemphasis on tracing how Āyurveda has been influenced by Greek elements. At the same time, he argued that there was strong Greek influence in the field of surgery, since the *Carakasamhita* and the Bower manuscript was devoid of surgical knowledge. At roughly the same time, between 1893 and 1912, A.F. Rudolf Hoernle, principal of the Calcutta Madrasa, undertook the editing and translation of the Bower manuscripts in Calcutta. He published a monograph on anatomical terms.[10] This study was a departure from the usual generalized descriptive commentaries. H.R. Zimmer looked at the mythical and allegorical elements in the Vedic and medical texts.[11] His acquaintance with C.G. Jung, the famous psychologist, created some interest in the psychological implications of mythology. Jean Filliozat, a French ophthalmologist by training with proficiency in Sanskrit and other Oriental and European classical languages, took up a comparative study of the development of medicinal doctrines in India.[12] He observed that Āyurveda is the legitimate heir to the Vedas but it has developed to a great extent the patrimony thus received. According to him, the Indian and Greek medical traditions had a parallel development. Before concluding this section, it has to be added that the contributions of Western scholars in general suffered from a lack of proficiency in understanding the original sources, which prevented them from arriving at correct conclusions regarding the nature and content of Indian medicine.

[10] A. F. Rudolf Hoernle, *Studies in the Medicine of Ancient India*, Part I: *Ostiology or the Bones of the Human Body* (Oxford: Oxford University Press, 1907).

[11] H.R. Zimmer, *Hindu Medicine* (Baltimore: Johns Hopkins University Press, 1948).

[12] Filliozat, *Classical Doctrines of Indian Medicines.*

The first Indian scholar to make an invaluable contribution to the study of ancient Indian medicine was G.N. Mukhopadhyaya Bishagacharya.[13] A product of the Calcutta Medical College, his work on surgical tools of ancient India is a brilliant study that provides valuable information about the instruments used by Āyurvedic physicians in surgery from ancient times. In addition to the description of tools based on Sanskrit texts, the scholar-physician compares the Indian instruments with those of the Greeks, Romans, Arabs, and the surgeons of modern medicine, with special emphasis on the variety and efficacy of the tools instead of culture-specific accounts of the earlier writings. Mukhopadhyaya, who was the chief editor of the *Journal of Āyurveda*, published in Calcutta from 1923 onwards, has several articles to his credit on various issues, including the status of Āyurveda in those days.[14]

Debiprasad Chattopadhyaya brought in a new element of sociological analysis and interpretation in the historiography of Āyurveda. He provides a critical sociological interpretation of medical science.[15] He emphasizes the need to undertake studies in sciences with reference to their socio-economic background. To him, science cannot be seen as an autonomous domain that is not influenced by society. This work establishes the idea of the development of a scientific methodology through the application of *yukti* (reason). Reasoning in the *Carakasamhita* testifies to the theoretical achievement of early Indian medicine. He maintains that a physician accomplished in rational application is always superior to one with mere empirical knowledge of these substances. At the same time, the author is unfortunately silent about the epigraphical sources that contain much valuable information for a sociological understanding of various aspects of medicine and its practice. Further, for all practical purposes, India meant British India for almost all the scholars who worked on various problems of history. Had he examined the epigraphic records, he

[13] G.N. Mukhopadhyaya Bishagacharya, *The Surgical Instruments of the Hindus*, 2 vols (Calcutta: Calcutta University Press, 1913–14); G.N. Mukhopadhyaya Bishagacharya, *History of Indian Medicine* 3 vols (Delhi: Orient Books Reprint Corporation, 1974).

[14] Bishagacharya, *History of Indian Medicine*, was published in three volumes in 1922–9.

[15] Debiprasad Chatoapadhyaya, *Science and Society in Ancient India* (Calcutta: Research India Publications, 1977).

would have seen that the geographical base of the science of Āyurveda was much wider than the British domain of the Indian subcontinent at least from the time of the Mauryan emperor Ashoka. The emperor declared in his Major Rock Edict II that he had made arrangements for two kinds of treatment, that is, treatment for humans and that for animals within his territories and outside it in the domains of the Yavanarāja of Antioch and his neighbouring regions. This means that the indigenous tradition of healing and healthcare had spread in those areas. This information seems to call for a reconsideration of the old issue of the so-called relation between the Indian and the Greek traditions of healthcare in the light of contact between the two domains of culture. However, for obvious reasons, we do not enter into that problem in the present context.

P.V. Sharma took his degree in Āyurveda from Banaras Hindu University and later served that university as the professor of *dravyaguna* (the medicinal qualities of herbs and other healing objects). A renowned scholar and physician, Sharma has contributed immensely to the study of pharmacology and the history of Āyurveda. His edited work, *History of Medicine in India from Antiquity to 1000 AD*, was published by the Indian National Science Academy. In Sharma's volume, there is an attempt to trace the development of ideas using the medical treatises and also from medical texts. Sharma has edited the classical text *Carakasamhita* with an English translation and this work is highly helpful for modern students to familiarize themselves with the original work in Āyurveda.[16] Sharma presents his balanced views on the dates of *Caraka* in the introduction to this volume.

G.U. Thite, an Indologist, published a work entitled *Medicine in Its Magico-religious Aspects According to the Vedic and Later Literature.* The author states that his main intention in the work was to study ancient Indian medicine not as a science but as a religious phenomenon.[17] However, it has been noted correctly that the work could not serve its aim due to several reasons, including the author's lack of proficiency in the Sanskrit language. Rahul Peter Das, in a

[16] P.V. Sharma, *Caraka Samhita*, Jai Krishna Ayurveda Series (Varanasi and Delhi: Chaukhamba Orientalia, 1981).

[17] G.U. Thite, *Medicine in Its Magico-religious Aspects According to the Vedic and Later Literature* (Poona: Continental Prakashan, 1982).

lengthy review article, has presented a scholarly critique of this work and has analysed the issue of magic, religion, and science in the context of medicine.[18] One can further delve into this, as observed by Kenneth G. Zysk, for a complete and careful examination and reappraisal of the issue against the modern scholarship in the history of medicine, religion, and anthropology.[19] The author has efficiently shown that the existence of empirical medicine is evident even at the time of the Rgvedic hymns.

Francis Zimmerman introduces a distinct approach in the study and interpretation of the science of Āyurveda.[20] His study uses the tools of bio-geography and linguistics for presenting an ecological reading of the three primary Sanskrit medical texts. This phase of historiography of Āyurveda witnessed some important and hitherto unknown aspects of the science of indigenous medicine. An attempt was made to explore other disciplines. Thus, Lallanji Gopal wrote about the beginnings of the hospital system in ancient India.[21] Similarly, S. Mahdi Hassan wrote on the relation between the ancient cultures and their medicinal traditions.[22]

Vijaya Deshpande has published an essay called 'Indian Influence on Early Chinese Ophthalmology: Glaucoma as a Case Study', in the *Bulletin of the School of Oriental and African Studies*.[23] The study, after making enquiries into Buddhist texts, observes that cataract surgery

[18] Rahul Peter Das, 'Review of Thite's *Medicine in Its Magico-religious Aspects According to the Vedic and Later Literature*', *Indo-Iranian Journal*, 1984, 27(3): 232–44.

[19] Kenneth G. Zysk, *Medicine in the Veda* (Delhi: Motilal Banarsidass Publishers Pvt. Ltd, 1998), 10.

[20] Francis Zimmerman, *The Jungle and the Aroma of Meats: An Ecological Theme in the Hindu Medicine* (Delhi: Motilal Banarsidass Publishers Pvt. Ltd., 1999).

[21] Lallanji Gopal, 'Beginnings of Hospital System in Ancient India', in *Vajapeya: Essays on Evolution of Indian Art and Culture*, ed. A.M. Sastri, R.K. Sarma, and A. Prasad, K.D. Bajpai Felicitation volumes, vol. 2 (Delhi: Abe Books, 1987).

[22] S. Mahdi Hassan, 'Alchemy and Its Fundamental Terms in Greek, Arabic, Sanskrit and Chinese', *Indian Journal of History of Science*, 1981, 16(1): 64–76.

[23] Vijaya Deshpande, 'Indian Influence on Early Chinese Ophthalmology: Glaucoma as a Case Study', *Bulletin of the School of Oriental and African Studies*, 1999, 62(2): 306–22.

was known to the surgeons prior to the composition of the *Uttaratantra* and that the dates of the composition of the text have to be pushed back in time to before the date of composition of that text, that is, earlier than the fourth century CE. According to the same authority, this is an idea expressed in the *Samyuktagama*, a Buddhist work generally attributed to the Jin dynasty of the period 350–431 CE.[24]

N.V.K. Varier was a practising physician, a social scientist, and a progressive scholar who approached the science of Āyurveda from a sociological point of view. Familiar with the original texts in Āyurveda, Varier was equipped with advanced knowledge in the subject. At the same time, wide reading and immense practical field experience made him well versed in the current politics of his time in addition to the knowledge of Āyurveda, both theoretical and practical. Aided by such a sense of history, he made a welcome attempt to interpret the underlying social and cultural meanings of the prevalent mythical and legendary accounts of the origin and early development of the science of Āyurveda.[25] Due to the nature of his studies, N.V.K. Varier had no opportunity to be familiar with the documents of earlier periods, and so he too was silent about the information contained in the epigraphic documents scattered over a vast area in the subcontinent. However, mention must be made about two sections on Aśvāyurveda (treatment of horses) and Vṛkṣāyurveda (treatment of trees and plants) in his volume, which contain valuable information about the material background of the science of indigenous medicine.

A much-welcome shift was brought in when a group of scholars moved away from the issues and problems regarding the antiquity of Āyurveda and also from the question of achievements of ancient Indian physicians. Instead, these new scholars emphasized the need for understanding the scientific developments that were taking place at various levels in society. Thus, Kenneth G. Zysk worked on some important issues, such as medicine in the Vedic hymns and the practices of healing in the Buddhist *vihāras* (monasteries). The medicinal tradition seen in the empirical framework of Āyurveda as found in the theoretical Samhita texts varied from the magico-religious tradition of

[24] V. Lilakrishnan, *Samyuktagama*, Malayalam Translation (Calicut: Prabhat Publishers, 2012), verse 39.

[25] N.V.K. Varier, *History of Āyurveda*, 56, Kottakal Ayurveda Series (Kottakkal: Arya Vaidya Sala, 2012).

the Vedas. Still, he finds the beginning of the emphasis on recording of observable facts in the Vedic hymns. He discusses in detail the problem of the Vedic origin of medicine in Āyurveda on the basis of medical references in the hymns of the *Rgveda* and the *Atharvaveda*. A large number of hymns are taken for analysis and textual annotation. Thus, the author takes the subject out of the conventional idea of myth and legends and into the actual scientific framework of categories of diseases, nature and content of medicine, and so forth. Thus, according to Zysk, the science of healing in the Vedas is not without a different approach to diseases and the tradition of healing.[26] The discussion as a whole makes it clear how the knowledge and practice of medicine underwent serious changes over the course of its growth over a long period.

Similarly, he has brought out a separate volume on Buddhist medicine.[27] Zysk observes, after examining several Buddhist texts of the *Nikayas* and *Piṭakas*, that the knowledge of anatomy developed in the *vihāras* when the *bhikṣus* (medicant saints) started acquiring objective knowledge of the internal organs of the human body through systematic observation and study.[28] The subject was dealt with by earlier scholars as cited above. Zysk analyses the topic of medicine in the monastery with reference to the Kuhnian concept of paradigm shift and finds that the concept is partly useful for analysing the issue but he observes that the monastic medicine retained some elements of tradition. However, he emphasizes the serious departures that were taking place in the science of Āyurveda when it was widely accepted as an effective mode of healing. Further, the basic Āyurvedic concepts, such as the *pañcabhūta* (five basic elements), *doṣa* (bodily humour), and so forth, are also in the focus of this work. Some portions show how the knowledge of anatomy originated and grew in the *vihāra*. Zysk's analysis of the topic shows that several ideas of the science of Āyurveda, taken as the foundation stone of the knowledge, appeared for the first time in the Buddhist monastery. In other words, the basic concepts of Āyurveda with several details found in the *samhithas* make their presence felt first in the Buddhist ideas, which are codified

[26] Zysk, *Medicine in the Veda*, 9–10.

[27] Kenneth G. Zysk, *Asceticism and Healing in Ancient India: Medicine in the Buddhist Monastery* (Delhi: Motilal Banarsidass Publishers Pvt. Ltd., 2000 [1991]).

[28] Zysk, *Asceticism and Healing in Ancient India*, 34–5.

in the Buddhist *Nikāyas* and *Piṭakas*. Zysk's study underlines the fact that enquiry into the science of Āyurveda would be incomplete without perusal of the Vedic hymns on the one side and the Buddhist texts on the other. Like many of the previous works, it has to be admitted that Zysk's approach to history often finds itself on slippery grounds. For example, his idea of the Vedic period as representing a monolithic culture would be a hindrance to tracing the changes that were taking place in Āyurveda within the long period of life of Vedic society. While appreciating the author's thorough command over the source material, it has to be mentioned that his view is myopic with respect to the differences between the earlier and later portions of Vedic literature. The result is that he missed the significant changes or shift of ideas that were occurring in the knowledge of diseases and their medicine in the hymns in the later portions of the *Rgveda* and the text of the *Atharvaveda*. Had he combined his data with some ideas about the chronology of the Vedic hymns, he would have been able to find that almost all of his information is from the first and the tenth *maṇḍalas* of the *Rgveda*, which are attributed to a later phase based on the lifestyle of the people. Here it may be noted that historians, such as R.S. Sharma have maintained that the six books from two to seven betray the features of an earlier epoch, while the books one, eight, nine, and ten represent a form of life which is different from that of the earlier-mentioned books. However, these blind spots do not minimize the value of Zysk's observations and formulations about Vedic and Buddhist knowledge of the indigenous science of medicine. A much welcome fund of information, the studies of Zysk provide access to the ideas contained in the ancient and medieval epigraphic sources with a special reference to the important aspects of management of diseases in religious institutions, such as the Buddhist monasteries and the Brahminical temples.

M.S. Valiathan, a well-known practising surgeon, who has done considerable research in Āyurvedic medicine, departs from many points in the conventional historiography of the subject.[29] His Legacy series (*Legacy of Caraka*, *Legacy of Suśruta*, and *Legacy of Vaghbhata*) provides detailed discussion and scholarly comments on the classical Indian texts of the science of Āyurveda. Valiathan observes that

[29] M.S. Valiathan, *An Introduction to Āyurveda* (Hyderabad: University Press, 2013).

Caraka's system of medicine had to be taken as more than a *tantra* or a manual of medicine, of which many were in existence. A system of medicine had to be built on philosophical foundations that would resist change, while the superstructure would undergo wear and tear and transformations over time. Living in an atmosphere charged with mutually contesting ideas, Caraka chose his 'foundation stones from different philosophical quarries and shaped them to suit the plan of his medical edifice'.[30] As pointed out by Das Gupta, Caraka's use of the evolution of the living being from the *Avyakta* identification of *Rajas* and *Tamas* with the aberrant state of mind and *Sattva* with the good represent the earliest systematic doctrine of *sāmkhya*. Caraka's extensive treatment of logical categories in relation to the Āyurvedic debate took place much before the codification of the *nyāya sūtras*. Caraka perhaps took the logical portion of the Samhita from earlier non-medical literature and incorporated them into his work. Valiathan discusses Caraka's selective approach to *Vaiśeṣika guṇas* in Chapter 1 of *The Legacy of Caraka*. He further notices that according to Caraka, medical knowledge existed in folklore, local health traditions, verbal testimony, and many other sources. The *Carakasamhita* according to Valiathan is a landmark and a creative revision of its forerunner, the *Agniveśatantra*.

Valiathan introduces Suśruta as a surgical colossus. He is of the opinion that the master of surgery preceded the great grammarian Panini. Based on events and persons of the Buddha's time, Valiathan takes Suśruta to a hoary past. Further, Valiathan observes that as suggested by Jyothirmitra, Kāśirāja Divodāsa had temporarily withdrawn to Bharadwaja's *āśrama* (hermitage) in Uttarakāśi following his defeat by the Haihaya Kṣatriyas, and the teaching of the *Suśrutatantra* had originated during his exile. He further maintains that the Samhita that bears Suśruta's name ranks with that of Caraka in authority and is a product of one or more redactions of an original *tantra*, which Suśruta had composed. Valiathan also discusses the process of the evolution of a *tantra* to a Samhita. Significantly, he underscores the fact that social changes had a major impact on the evolution of the *Suśrutasamhita*. According to him, the redaction of *Suśrutatantra* into the present *Suśrutasamhita* took place after Caraka's transformation of the *Agniveśatantra* into the *Carakasamhita*. Valiathan also

[30] Raghava Varier, *Charaka: Intellectual Background* (Kottakkal: Arya Vaidya Sala, 2001), 23–8.

discusses the philosophical and semantic aspects of the medical vision of the great master of the Indian surgical tradition.

Valiathan writes in his *The Legacy of Suśruta* that Suśruta's surgical procedures had more or less disappeared from the mainstream of Āyurvedic practice after Vāgbhaṭa and had survived precariously in the hands of traditional practitioners. The technology for surgical instrumentation faded away, 'unwept and unsung'. Surgery had no more masters and schools and the old techniques survived only in the hands of itinerant practitioners.[31] Quite contrary to this statement, there are numerous documents scattered over a vast area in the northern and southern parts of India referring to provisions including *āturaśālais* (health centres) and infrastructural facilities for treatment, including physicians, surgeons, nurses, service personnel, and so forth. They were provided with landed property and remuneration in cash for the services rendered by them. According to Valiathan, what is important about Vāgbhaṭa is the emphasis given to the practical aspects of treatment. Vāgbhaṭa's identity, nativity, date, and so on are still subjects of controversy. While the concept of *pañcabhūta*, a cornerstone of Āyurveda, received serious and illuminating attention from Caraka, *Aṣṭāṅgasaṅgraha* and *Aṣṭāṅgahṛdaya* skipped such topics and the related questions of *prakṛti* (basic nature) and *puruṣa* (functioning self) and the homology of the human microcosm and the universal macrocosm. Here the author rightly observes that healthcare became more of a practical art with decreasing emphasis on its philosophical emphasis due probably to the evolution of the medicine after Caraka.

Another observation of Valiathan is that several stages of continuity and change took place in the ancient Indian medical practice over the course of several centuries that intervened between the *Atharvaveda* and the *Carakasamhita*. He gives due importance to the valuable contributions of Buddhist monasteries not only in promoting the cause of Āyurveda but also in providing a strong empirical, rational, and philosophical base for the science of healing in ancient India. Healing in the Vedas, medicine in monasteries, and the later composition of Vāgbhaṭa mark the major watersheds of this system of knowledge. True to the spirit of the Indian civilization, tradition and modernity are not mutually exclusive categories, just as in the tradition

[31] M.S. Valiathan, *The Legacy of Suśruta* (Hyderabad: University Press, 2013), 6.

of the scientific system of Āyurveda. Therefore, a total and subversive shift of paradigm is almost out of the question in the tradition of Indian medicine. Every aspect of tradition is endowed with a point of modernity, which tends to proceed further. Similarly, the spirit of modernity is always built on the firm base of a tradition. The elements of continuity and change are long processes in the knowledge of Āyurveda as in any other Indian systems of knowledge. However, Valiathan does not make any attempt to place the developments in their historical background.

I concur with Valiathan wholeheartedly in his observation that there are numerous possibilities for applying basic science to investigate a whole range of concepts, procedures, and products, which are important in the theory and practice of Āyurveda. The investigation would be based on the methods of physiology, immunology, cell biology, molecular biology, bio-organic chemistry, and allied branches of science, and would be just as rigorous, but their clues in the new approach would always be drawn from Āyurveda. As the studies ramify and accumulate novel, useful, and interesting findings, they would create the prospect of a new discipline—Āyurvedic biology—which would look at diverse problems ranging from phenotype correlation of populations to the effect of traditional formulations on mitochondrial function or the repair of breaks in the DNA chain.[32] Āyurvedic biology would represent new sprouts in the age-old tree of Āyurveda, which never failed to interest modern science since the East–West encounter began in India centuries ago.

By way of concluding this section, it may be stated that recently there has begun a new trend that has brought to light a rich fund of sources in the form of epigraphic documents scattered over a vast area of the Indian subcontinent. Thus, Niranjana Devi examines the social developments in the practice of Āyurveda in medieval South India.[33] Referring to a number of medieval inscriptions in the temples of Tamil Nadu, Devi presents interesting details of the practices of Āyurvedic physicians and surgeons in the rural villages of Tamil Nadu during the period under consideration. She has worked a lot on collecting details about health centres, medicines prepared in the *ātulasālai* (hospital), status of the personnel who were engaged in the profession, remuneration for various posts in the medical profession,

[32] Valiathan, *An Introduction to Āyurveda*, 140.

[33] R. Niranjana, *Medicine in South India* (Chennai: Eswar Press, 2004).

and so on. At the same time, it has to be admitted that Devi has not been able to explain the developments in their social, economic, and historical context. Still, the rich data presented by her for future researchers of the subject remain invaluable.

In a recent volume, Susmita Basu Majumdar and Nayana Sharma Mukherjee have culled out a rich corpus of interesting information from epigraphic documents about medical practitioners, medical institutions, and the medicines that were used in healthcare centres in different parts of the country.[34] In the preface to their volume, Majumdar and Mukherjee have gratifyingly referred to the importance of inscriptional data as a treasure trove of immensely valuable information. In the first chapter of this volume, they have consulted a large number of available epigraphic records, including the label inscriptions of some Buddhist sites in various parts of the subcontinent for understanding various issues of the topic. This helped them furnish useful data for obtaining information about the social status of physicians, functioning of hospitals, and the preparation and storage of medicines in different parts of the country in general and southern India in particular. In addition to these, Majumdar and Mukherjee have paid some attention to the historical evolution of the practice, not only of medicine but also surgical treatment, including rhinoplasty in ancient and medieval epochs of Indian history. One chapter in Majumdar and Mukherjee's volume pays special attention to ophthalmology in the *Uttaratantra* of the Samhita. Here, they bring out interesting details about the knowledge and method of the surgical procedure in particular. The sections on the anatomical description of the eye, refractive errors, conjunctivitis, glaucoma, cataract surgery, and so on are also highly useful not only for general readers but also for students and researchers of Āyurveda. In another essay in the volume, Majumdar and Mukherjee provide interesting aspects of rhinoplasty, an Indian surgical procedure.[35] This is of great importance in the history of indigenous traditions of surgical treatment in that 'it led to the discovery by the West of a particular procedure of nasal reconstruction that gave India her deserving position in the annals of plastic surgery, especially in the field of rhinoplasty, and is

[34] Susmita B. Majumdar and Nayana S. Mukherjee, *Essays on History of Medicine* (Mumbai: Indian Institute of Research in Numismatic Studies [IIRNS], 2013).

[35] Majumdar and Mukherjee, *Essays on History of Medicine.*

still known as "the Indian method"'.[36] The subject matter of another essay in this collection is the invaluable pieces of information regarding the indigenous tradition of surgical operations.[37] The tables attached to the essay on the services of two surgeons of the nineteenth century is highly informative in social, historical, and scientific aspects. It is clear from the tables that a large number of the patients were women. Out of one hundred cases, 63 were of female patients. The amputation of the nose was a social malaise in India, which was used as a means of settling personal grudges, and a punitive measure for misdeeds, misbehaviour, as well as violation of the sanctity of marriage. A brief survey of the studies on the history of Indian medicine given in this anthology will be very useful for those who are interested in the subject.

Similarly, an essay by Ranbir Chakravarty and Krishnendu Ray makes an enquiry into the details about healing houses, physicians, various uses of medicine, and therapeutic strategies by referring to the available epigraphic sources, mainly from the medieval Indian regional communities.[38] The essay starts with a brief critique of the conceptual apparatus of the existing knowledge of ancient Indian medicine. Further, there is an attempt to place the available data in its historical context. However, there are interesting materials waiting for a proper perspective-based and historical explanation with reference to the social context to which they belong. It is gratifying that more and more scholars are engaged in the epigraphic sources, which were neglected by earlier scholars working on the history of Āyurveda.

[36] Majumdar and Mukherjee, *Essays on History of Medicine*, 67–88.

[37] Majumdar and Mukherjee, *Essays on History of Medicine*, 53–65.

[38] Ranbir Chakravarty and Krishnendu Ray, *Healing and Healers Inscribed: Epigraphic Bearings on Healing Houses in Early India*, Occasional Paper 30 (Kolkata: Institute of Development Studies, 2011).

1

Early Historic Phase

Indus Civilization: Traditions of Healing

An enquiry into the Indian tradition of healing and healthcare has to be traced back to the proto-historic Harappan culture, which is attributed to a period from c. 2300 to 1700 BCE, contemporaneous with the old civilizations of Egypt, Sumer, Akkad, Mesopotamia, and so forth. Innumerable sites, scattered over the vast area comprising the modern countries of India and Pakistan, yielded a large variety of materials pertaining to the economy, society, and culture of this civilization. The main sources of information for this phase of Indian civilization are excavated materials, including remains of urban sites, big tanks, tools, implements, and a large number of inscribed seals from various Harappan sites in the subcontinent.[1] The inscriptions on the seals have not been convincingly deciphered so far due to the fact that both the script and the language used in the writings are unknown till date. The pieces of information, therefore, are speculative in nature. However, they are valuable in the absence of other tangible evidences.

[1] For a general account of the subject and for some photographic plates, see Sir Mortimer Wheeler, *The Indus Civilization*, 3rd Edition (Cambridge: Cambridge University Press, 1968).

Information about the healing tradition of the Harappan people is very scanty and fragmented. Herbal medicines were used by all the old-world cultures and, therefore, it is not improbable that the people of the Indus Valley also had some knowledge of the medicinal value of plants and simples as suggested by scholars (see, for example, R. Niranjana's *Medicine in South India*). It seems to be important in this context to mention the worship of plants, which is a recurring motif in several of the Indus seals. This has been understood as an indication of the popularity of the worship of herbal plants thought to be probably endowed with fertility and magical powers. This is supported by several seals yielded by various Harappan sites.[2] If this is correct, the continuity of this can be traced in the Vedic culture, which considered a large number of plants as medicines. It is interesting to note in this connection that scholars, such as D.D. Kosambi, have considered this continuity of cultures of this type to be a characteristic feature of Indian civilization.[3] The proto-historic tradition of India also has this motif of plant worship among several other signs as found on the Indus seals.[4]

Scholars have suggested, on the basis of materials from the trenches, that water, the central purifying agent, was considered an important medicine during the period of the Indus civilization. It is highly probable that treatment by water was a therapeutic measure practiced by the Indus people to restore and preserve health.[5] A black ball-like object received from an Indus site was recognized by archaeologists as asphalt (*shilajit* or *kanmada*), a secretion of stone. A recent scholar-historian of Āyurveda argues, not without reason, that this must have been brought down to the Indus Valley for medicinal use, especially for treatment of disorders in the urinary tract.[6] The occurrence of *shilajit* as well as arsenic, coral stag,

[2] Asko Parpola, *Deciphering the Indus Script*, paperback edition (Delhi: Cambridge University Press, 2000), 109. See also Fr. Heras, *Studies in Proto-Indo-Mediterranean Culture* (Bombay: Indian Historical Research Institute, St Xavier's College, 1953), 229.

[3] D.D. Kosambi, *Culture and Civilization of Ancient India in Historic Outline* (London: Routledge and Kegan Paul, 1965).

[4] M.R. Raghava Varier, 'The Edakal Engravings Revisited', in *Kerala Archaeological Series* (*KAS*), 2001, I: 34–7.

[5] Zysk, *Medicine in the Veda*, 2.

[6] Varier, *History of Āyurveda*, 20.

and rhinoceros horn at Mohenjo-Daro leads us to the conclusion that those objects had acquired a reputation as powerful objects having medicinal value in the proto-historic period and they were known since the Harappan times for their medicinal qualities. Scholars and historians are of the opinion that some sort of surgical technique of trepanation had been practised during the Harappan times. A skull (H 796 B) from the cemetery R 37, Harappa, has reportedly a hole in the tempero-paretal region, and this is taken by some to suggest an opening made for trepanation. The skull of a child, found in a trench at Kalibangan, with three holes on the right side is also interesting. The wounds show signs of healing and it is argued that the child must have survived surgical operation.[7] The discoveries of a vast range of copper objects, such as knives, needles, borers, and chisels probably used for some surgical purposes, become suggestive in the context of these observations.[8]

Scholars and historians are divided on the issue of the end of the Indus civilization. Some scholars, such as Sir Mortimer Wheeler, are of the opinion that the civilization disappeared totally somewhere in the first quarter of the second millennium BCE, while others, such as Romila Thapar, hold that a meaningful mixture of elements of the Harappan culture into the emerging Vedic society took place as suggested by evidence brought to light relatively recently. The data which formed the basis for arguing for this aspect of continuity of the Indus culture is in the form of pottery yielded by a number of sites, such as Bhagawanpura in the Kurukshetra district, Dadheri in Ludhiana, Katpalan and Nagar in the Jalandhar district, and Manda in Jammu.[9]

[7] Zysk, *Medicine in the Veda*, 3–4. For photos of the skulls from Harappa #H796/B and Kalibangan #KLB 8/69, see Zysk, *Medicine in the Veda*, 209. See also Amiya K. Roy Choudhury, 'Trepanation in Ancient India', *Asiatic Society of Calcutta*, 1972, 25: 203–6.

[8] Ernest Mackay quoted in M.N. Deshpande, 'Archaeological Sources for the Reconstruction of the History of Sciences of India', *Indian Journal of History of Science*, 1971, 6(1): 13.

[9] Jagat Pati Joshi and Madhubala, 'Life during the Period of Overlap of late Harappa and PGW Cultures', *Journal of the Indian Society of Oriental Art*, Dr Moti Chandra Commemoration Volume, Part II, 1977–8, IX: 20–9. See also R.S. Sharma, *Material Culture and Social Formations in Ancient India* (Delhi: MacMillan, 1983), 23.

Vedic Society: The Historical Setting

The main source for understanding the socio-economic and cultural developments in the Vedic society is the corpus of the Ȑgvedic hymns. Generally, the entire collection of hymns, including those in the *Atharvaveda*, are taken to represent a single social formation, that is, the Vedic society.[10] It has been convincingly shown that even the corpus of hymns in the *Ȑgveda* represents not a single phase but at least two separate stages of social formation. According to this view, the *maṇḍalas* from the II to VII, called the Family Books, are considered the earliest portions, which show features of an earlier social formation belonging approximately to a period from c. 1500 to 1000 BCE. Rgvedic society in this early phase was predominantly pastoral, though agriculture was not totally unknown. Cattle was a form of property and, therefore, cattle raids and battles for recapturing stolen cattle were perpetual events. There are several terms derived from *go*, meaning cattle, such as *gaviṣṭi, gaveṣaṇa, goṣu, gavyat, gavyu,* and so on, all meaning war. Predominantly tribal in nature, war was a natural and logical economic function in Rgvedic society.[11] War was also recognized as a legitimate mode of livelihood in the *Dharmaśāstras* of the later period. The perpetual conflicts and war for cattle most probably account for the repeated references to broken limbs, injuries, and so forth in the Ȑgvedic hymns. The hymns in this portion have only sporadic and scanty references to diseases and the treatment for them. What is mainly available in this portion are medicines that are rudimentary and very simple. Water is referred to as a healing agent in one of the hymns.

It is interesting to note that a large number of references are made in the Ȑgvedic hymns to treatments for supposedly fatal wounds. Stories are told of how the sage Dīrghatamas was cut into pieces by his enemies and how the twin-god Aśvinidevas, the celestial physicians, gave him life by joining together the parts of his body; how Visphala, the wife of Khelarāja, lost her legs in the battlefield and how a metallic leg was grafted;[12] how Śyāvāśva was cut into pieces and then got back his life; how the sage Atri's severed limbs were grafted; how Dadhici's head was cut off and replaced shortly with a

[10] See, for example, Zysk, *Medicine in the Veda*, 129.

[11] Sharma, *Material Culture*, 24, 38.

[12] *Rgveda* 1: 115–16

horse's head and then later re-grafted once again to his body, and so on.[13] The meaning and significance of these stories of amputation and grafting become clear when they are placed in their historical contexts.

Recurring attempts to increase cattle wealth and to protect it from enemies resulted in frequent inter-tribal conflicts. These conflicts were on the level of an economic activity and so every able-bodied member of the group was expected to take part in the fighting. This seems to explain why heroism and prowess in warfare were eulogized in several contexts in the Vedic mantras. Sometimes, these fights led to a large number of casualties. It is in this historical context that the repeated references to amputation and grafting of limbs become meaningful. However, these references need not be taken to reflect a social reality; nor are they taken to be comparable with modern surgical processes. In all probability they are derived mostly from poetic imagination and from the exaggeration that is possible in a heroic world with a fund of mythic lore.

The Eastward Migration of the Vedic People

A major historical process that had far-reaching effects in the society, economy, and culture of the period under discussion was the eastward migration of the Vedic people and the long process of their settling in the Ganga–Yamuna valley up to the eastern parts of present-day Uttar Pradesh and Bihar. Clear-felling of the thick forests of the Gangetic basin on a large scale was crucial in this migration, for which iron tools and implements were essential. Numerous excavated sites in the region and a variety of iron objects recovered from those sites gain importance in the context of these historical developments. Needless to say, tremendous changes were taking place in Vedic society during the period represented, especially in the later Vedic texts, including books one and ten of the *Rgveda*, the hymns of the *Atharvaveda*, and the Brāhmaṇas. In the *Śatapatha Brāhmaṇa*, there is a story which is taken by historians, such as D.D. Kosambi, to be a representation of the eastward migration of the Vedic people from the Punjab region. According to the text, Māthava, the king of Videgha, was performing a great *yajña* (Vedic ritual) on the bank of the river

[13] *Rgveda* 1: 110–12.

Sarasvati, with Gotama Rahūgaṇa as the chief priest. Agni Vaiśvānara, the Vedic god who was in the mouth of the chief priest Gotama Rahūgaṇa, jumped out of his mouth and walked eastward. King Videgha Māthava and the priest Gōtama Rahūgaṇa followed the God Agni, who walked for long to the east, finally crossed the river Sadānīra, the modern Gaṇḍak, and stopped there. Agni Vaiśvānara told Videgha Māthava and Gōtama Rahūgaṇa: 'I have not tasted this region so far. Hereafter you perform your *yajña* here.' Thereafter, they continued the ritual in the new region. This is evidently a story that relates the spread of the *yajña* ritual and the Vedic society upto the regions of eastern Uttar Pradesh and Bihar.[14] The hostile natural surroundings and the unfamiliar weather and climate in addition to the hard work were sufficient for causing a variety of ailments both external and internal, for which some kind of remedy was essential. It is only logical to surmise that as the Vedic society existed in such a situation for long, it must have accumulated some sort of knowledge of corrective measures for escaping from diseases.

Historical Developments

Efficient plough agriculture with an iron ploughshare began in the region around 600 BCE as shown by the archaeological artefacts yielded by stratified trenches. The prolific use of an iron axe, spade, sickle, and similar tools and implements were highly useful in clearing the thick forests of the Ganga valley. This was, in all probability, the result of large-scale human settlements in this region. More and more land was brought under the plough and this resulted in the spread of agriculture into new areas. Contemporary sources, including the later Vedic hymns and sources such as the *Āraṇyakas* and the *Brāmaṇas* mention several new lentils, pulses, and peas that were grown in the regions, which indicates some new trends in the food habits of common people. Significantly, the Āyurvedic texts contain references to the nature of ingredients of those foodgrains and their resultant effects on the human physical system.

Increase in agriculture led to the production of surplus and this prepared ground for the rise and growth of urban settlements in the

[14] D.D. Kosambi, *An Introduction to the Study of Indian History* (Bombay: Popular Prakasan, 1975), 123.

north-eastern parts of India around 600 BCE. As many as 20 *nagaras* (town) are mentioned by their names in the Buddhist Pāli texts. These literary references are profoundly supported and complemented by the excavated materials from a large number of sites in the Ganga–Yamuna doab. Certain features of town life as suggested by our sources are relevant in the historical context of healthcare. Eating houses[15] were becoming more and more familiar features of the urban life. The Brahminical attitude to this trend was not friendly but the Buddhists were accepting. The trend was so powerful that even the Brahminical sections were not able to keep away from the 'order of the day'. The *Āpastamba Dharmasūtra* advises higher classes not to eat food prepared in shops, but some items are exempted from this restriction.

Archaeological evidence shows that this phase of the towns was at its peak during the Kuṣāṇa period. Mathura (Sonkh) has yielded as many as seven layers of Kuṣāṇa structures, while the Gupta remains were only one or two. This is important because the Kuṣāṇa period is closely connected with the final redaction of the *Carakasamhita*, one of the basic texts of medicine, and also because the text has some portions which show links with the needs of pleasure seeking and an elitist urban population. The modes of treatment, such as *rasāyana* (rejuvenation) and *vājīkaraṇa* (aphrodisiacs), become relevant in such a historical background.

Development and Diseases

The developments discussed above were the sources of several diseases and acute problems of health. For example, the growth and developments of trade routes and the long and hazardous journeys through them created several health problems. A major issue was the resisting of natural urges for a long time during the journeys, which is considered to be the root cause of several ailments.

The formation of the state and the resultant emergence of local kingdoms in the *Janapadas* (human settlement) led to rivalries constantly developing among them, mainly due to the insufficiency of resources. Mutual conflicts and warfare were regular events. This

15 Eating houses were places along the trade routes where food was available.

seems to explain the need for physicians and surgeons, as mentioned in the *Suśrutasamhita*, to remove objects, such as arrows and so forth, from the body of soldiers and the treatment of wounds so inflicted. The development of a whole branch of treatment known as *śalyacikitsa* (surgery) acquires significance in this historical context. Interestingly enough, there is a long section in the *Suśrutasamhita* on military science. The use of poisons in political relations was common in those days as mentioned in Kautalya's *Arthaśāstra* and this explains the presence of a section on *agada tantra* (toxicology) in the *Suśrutasamhita*.[16] It has to be noted in this connection that a knowledge of developments in the areas of economic, social, and political history is essential for understanding the nature and content of medicine and its practice.

Early History: The Art of Healing in Vedic Texts

The earliest source of information to trace the history of indigenous knowledge of healing and healthcare is the corpus of the Rgvedic hymns, which is dated c. 1500–600 BCE. The conventional historiography of Āyurveda considers the entire corpus of the 1,017 hymns as a monolithic text but it has been convincingly shown, as we have noted, that books two to seven belong to an earlier stage of society whereas books one, eight, nine, and ten show the features of social formation of a later stage.[17] This later layer is dated on the basis of the social formation represented in it, to a period between 1000 and 600 BCE. A hymn in the *Rgveda* describes medicinal herbs as 'kings in their councils'.[18] This hymn could be composed only in a society in which formation of the state, at least in its primary form, must have taken place. Such a state appeared for the first time in India during the period of the *Janapada*s, c. 800–600 BCE, as shown by historians, such as Romila Thapar, R.S. Sharma, and A.L. Basham.[19]

Significantly enough, most of the references to the art of healing and the use of various medicines are found in books one and ten of the *Rgveda* and to a much greater extent in the hymns of the *Atharvaveda*

[16] See the chapter on *Suśrutasamhita*.

[17] Sharma, *Material Culture*, 36–7.

[18] *Rgveda* 10, 9: 7–20.

[19] Sharma, *Material Culture*, 166.

and the passages in the Brāhmaṇas, thereby suggesting that the earliest recorded history of medicine in India has to be traced to the period in which these texts were written. There are several hymns in the later *maṇḍalas* of the *Rgveda* and the other texts, which provide either simply the names of diseases or details of the ailments. Thus, we hear about several diseases, such as *amīva* (pain), *ascites* (water-belly, probably the disease *mahodara*), *balāsa* (swelling), *hariman* (jaundice), *hridroga* (probably chest pain), *jvara* (fever), *kāsa* (cough), *kilāsa* (leuko-derma), *kṛmi* (worms), *rapas* (deformity and swelling of limbs), *takman* (malaria), *unmāda* (insanity), *viṣkandha* (tetanus), *yakṣma* (tuberculosis), loss of blood, constipation, retention of urine, broken limbs, flesh wounds, and so forth.[20] *Aithareya Brāhmaṇa* 1, 4: 8 refers to diseases like *gaṇḍamāla* (goitre). One of them relates how Aśvinidevas rejuvenated Cyavana and Vandana in their old age (1, 116: 10). Ȅjvaśva and Kaṇva gained eyesight thanks to the treatment of the celestial physicians (1, 116: 16). Vadhrimati, wife of a eunuch, was blessed with an offspring (1, 116: 13). A close look at the list would show that some of the above-mentioned sicknesses are complicated and internal, whereas some are external and accidental. The list becomes meaningful only against its historical background.

Later Vedic Literature: The Brāhmaṇas

Equally relevant are the *Atharvaveda* and the Brāhmaṇas, especially the *Aithareya Brāhmaṇa* and the *Śatapatha Brāhmaṇa*, which are taken to form a part of the later Vedic texts. More and more details about medicine, treatment, and physicians are available in the Brāhmaṇa texts, especially in the *Aithareya Brāhmaṇa* and the *Śatapatha Brāhmaṇa*. A healing powder of natural elements is mentioned in several hymns. Thus, according to the *Aithareya Brāhmaṇa* (1: 52), fire or heat is the medicine to restore life. Soma is regarded as the king of creepers and medicinal plants. Nature cure, that is, the treatment with the aid of natural elements such as water, air, heat, and earth, was the main mode of treatment in the early Vedic age. The *Aithareya Brāhmaṇa* (8, 37: 4) makes a categorical observation that rainwater charged with the rays of the sun is a medicinal or potent drink. Vedic seers appear to have had some knowledge of toxicology. They knew that tamarind,

[20] For a detailed account, see Zysk, *Medicine in the Veda*, 12–89.

curd, and similar drinks neutralize the ill-effects caused by toxic drinks and drugs. The same text records how Mitra and Varuṇa, two Vedic gods, neutralized the effect of toxicants with curd.

Knowledge of Anatomy

According to the procedure of the *yajña* ritual, as shown by the later Vedic texts, it was obligatory on the part of the priests to utter the name of the part of the body as it was cut and offered to the deity. This is the content of a hymn in the *Rgveda* and this was to be followed in the case of human sacrifices too, as specified by later tradition. It has been observed that fairly accurate lists of anatomical parts of the human body and of horses have been preserved and transmitted through the texts of the Brāhmaṇas.[21] These texts are tentatively attributed to a period from the eighth to the fifth century BCE. This seems to suggest an earlier date for the ancient Indian knowledge of human anatomy when compared to that of Western culture. However, several of the parts were left unidentified since their names were in the local languages. Sometimes, they were only a portion of a bigger part. It is in the Samhitas that we get fuller and more advanced knowledge, thanks to a visual inspection of the human body and a method of dissection, which became part of the medical education, thus contributing substantially to the understanding of the human body.

A more advanced knowledge of diseases and their treatments is found in the *Atharvaveda*, which represents a relatively developed phase of social formation. Medicines and their uses in specific diseases are mentioned in several contexts. During this period there was considerable advancement in the knowledge of the human anatomy. There are descriptions of parts of the human body, such as arteries and veins, bones, marrow, flesh, joints, skin, breasts, eyes, nose, and teeth. The use of a catheter for releasing urine and certain apparatus for the opening of boils are mentioned. The treatment for poisoning is also described. Repeated references in the form of descriptive statements, prescriptive directions, and allusions to diseases, medicines,

[21] Zysk, *Medicine in the Veda*, 7. See also his article, 'The Evolution of Anatomical Knowledge in Ancient India, with Special Reference to Cross-Cultural influences', *Journal of African and Oriental Studies*, 106 (4): 1986, 687–705.

context of medicine. Close reading and proper understanding of the meaning of hymns in the *Rgveda* prove that plants and herbs were put under rigorous scrutiny and their important features and qualities were noted. This technique of recording valuable facts illustrates the very beginning of the empirical mode of thought. As suggested by a recent authority, this may be seen as 'the very beginning of the Indian's empirical mode of thought'.[23]

According to the clear information culled out from our sources, it is evident that there existed some kind of classificatory system of thinking.[24] The technique of diagnosis and prognosis illustrates the importance given to the recording of observable facts. Significantly enough, Vedic healing involved both the medicinal practice and a form of surgery. For example, in the treatment of the retention of urine, a reed was used as a catheter. Cauterization with caustic medicines was in vogue. Sand was in use in order to stop the flow of blood from the uterus or from a wound. It is known from the hymns that some kind of resin was applied to wounds for preventing them from bleeding and also to aid in the process of healing. Ointments and dyes were applied to the skin and a certain plant was in use for promoting the growth of hair. Water was a medicine used for the treatment of several diseases, both internal and external.

The Atharvavedic hymns speak of the instinctive use of medicinal plants by animals, such as cows, sheep, goats, eagles, serpents, porcupines (8, 7: 23–6), and so on. This need not be a new invention of Vedic society. As we have noted above, at least some knowledge of the medicinal qualities of herbs was, in all probability, inherited from the preceding cultures, especially the Indus culture that had some idea of the 'divine qualities' of plants as suggested by some motifs on the Indus seals. However, this has to be supported by further evidences to make any definite statement about this aspect.

A large number of physicians and medicinal plants (2, 9: 3) find mention in the texts. Thus, Brahma, Indra, Surya, and Aśvinidevas are referred to as celestial physicians, probably extending the human social experience of the art of healing to the celestial realm too. It has been noted earlier that the *Atharvaveda* referring to medicine and physicians is an indication of a considerable awareness of prevailing medical knowledge and practice at that time. The medical references

23 Zysk, *Medicine in the Veda*, 9.

24 Zysk, *Medicine in the Veda*, 12–17.

in the *Atharvaveda* can thus be taken to reflect a pre-existing body of ancient traditional knowledge that prevailed in pre-Vedic societies. The great *ācāryas* (perceptors), such as Caraka and Suśruta themselves, have stated that the roots of that knowledge lay in the older tradition of pre-Vedic society, which was largely nomadic, tribal, and pastoral. Thus, it can be convincingly argued that the *Atharvaveda* hymns set the basis for a systematic knowledge of prevention and cure of diseases, the use of medicinal herbs, the preparation and procedures of formulations, and so forth. It can also be held that the science of Āyurveda derives its authority and status, to begin with, from the *Atharvaveda* tradition of Vedic society and culture.

The hymns in the *Atharvaveda* mention nearly a hundred major and minor ailments and it is significant to note that these are classified in the verses 9, 8: 1–21 as those affecting the head, heart, abdomen, back, rectum, blood, limbs, and bones. There are references to general diseases too. Along with these, there are references to about 100 medicinal plants by their name. Incantations and rituals are over and above the use of medicinal plants. This seems to imply that the therapeutic principle here appears to have been established on a firm ground of rationale of a psycho somatic approach to the treatment of such diseases. It has been reasonably argued recently that this approach prevails even today with common people and perhaps in modern medical practice in the form of a 'placebo'.[25] In this context, it is important to note that these remedies are often used as supplements to the prescription of regular medicines. The incantations of hymns gave these medicinal formulations a Vedic authority. Thus, it can also be noted in many of the cases that the Vedic rishis had practical knowledge not only of human anatomy but of human psychology too.

Atharvaveda 3: 1 is a specific instance of surgical intervention accompanied by an incantation. From the hymns it can be gathered that the therapeutic strategy included some techniques like the catheter. This was used in the case of urinary troubles for removing the blockage of urine. A wide range and type of highly interesting problems relating to poisons, such as snake bites, scorpion stings, poison by enemies, and so forth, are addressed in the hymns. It has to be noted that the role of the mind was important in the context of a variety of problems of health.

[25] N. Krishnaswamy, *Āyurveda For the First-Time Reader* (Chennai: Vidyaprakash Publication, 2013), 12.

Medicine in the Brāhmaṇas includes *ōṣadhi* and *vīrudh* (creepers) that may be taken to come from the earth. Empirical knowledge in and experience with the properties of flora in the native region led to the development of a rich pharmacopoeia.[26] Medicines were either collected from the surrounding areas or brought from distant places and traded. What is significant in this is that many of the medicines are said to be brought from distant places. For example, *kuśṭha*, a remedy for a variety of diseases, grows in the mountainous regions and, therefore, had to be brought from distant places and traded, while *gulgulu* came from abroad by sea. The mode of acquisition of such medicines unmistakably points to the spread of trade and trading centres. Significantly, these statements are met with in those hymns (*Atharvaveda* 19, 38: 2), which are to be attributed to the period of urban development in the Ganga–Yamuna valley. The growth of towns towards the end of this phase can be presumed from the use of several terms, such as *nagara*, *nagarin* (town-dweller), and so on, in the texts of this period. In addition to this, these texts mention the names of Kauśambi, Kosala, and Vidarbha as big towns. Excavated sites support this view by yielding relics, which prove the existence of three urban centres, Ahicchatra, Kauśāmbi, and Hastinapura. The origin and growth of these centres are attributed by experts and historians to the sixth century BCE.[27]

An integral part of the acquisition of medicinal plants was the exact knowledge of them. Some kind of primitive system of classification that was based on gross morphology is fully praised by both the later-written books in the *Rgveda* and by the *Atharvaveda*. Plants thus collected were changed into medicine either by dicoction or by concoction. Sometimes they were used for making amulets. The healer knew the mode of preparation of the medicine. The later *maṇḍalas* of the *Rgveda* and the *Atharvaveda* mention the names of about 64 herbal plants that were in use as medicine.[28]

The origin and transmission of the knowledge of these herbal medicines cannot be explained easily. It must have been inherited

[26] Jogiraj Basu, *India of the Age of the Brahmanas* (Calcutta: Sanskrit Pustaka Bhandar, 1969), 64–5.

[27] R.S. Sharma, *Perspectives in Social and Economic History of Early India* (Delhi: Munshiram Manoharlal, 1983), 116–17.

[28] Zysk, *Medicine in the Veda* (Delhi: Motilal Benarsidass, 1998, 2nd edition), 10–11, 257–60.

from an earlier period. However, *virya*, the strength, and *rasa*, the essence of medicines, were known and there was some kind of classification of these qualities: *rasa* and *virya*. One of the hymns in the tenth *maṇḍala* of the *Rgveda* describes the healer as *vipro medhavi rasavīryabhāvanābhijño*, referring to the healer who is aware of the qualities of medicine. They are:

> *Rasa*, taste,
> *Guṇa*, quality,
> *Vīrya*, potency,
> *Vipāka*, effect of transformation, and
> *Prabhāva*, the curative power, that is, capability.

When we come to the later *maṇḍalas* we hear about new diseases. Hostile geographical surroundings in the newly reclaimed areas coupled with the unfriendly climate must have been the cause of several illnesses, especially of *takman* (malaria). *Jalaṣa*, or Rudra's medicine, is prescribed for 'Rudra's disease'. The exact meaning of the name of this drug is not clear. We know it is a liquid since, in one context, the instruction is to sprinkle it on the affected areas of the body (*Atharvaveda*, 6, 57: 2). In certain instances, it has been referred to as Rudra's *mūtra* (urine). It may be remembered here that urine, mainly from animals, is a medicine in Āyurveda.

The nomenclature of the ailments seems to indicate at least a primary level of categorization of diseases, mainly based on the areas affected or even pertaining to the mode of manifestation. The mantras do not indicate any causal explanation for ailments other than the wrath of demons or evil spirits. These ailments are attributed generally to the wrath of spirits and, therefore, their treatment involves the appeasement of the demons. Hence, Vedic medicine is described as magico-religious. A recent scholar has understood this fact differently: as a therapeutic approach that 'prevails even today with common people and perhaps in the modern medical practice in the garb of placebos'.[29] These remedies are often used as supplements to the prescription of regular medicines and the foregoing survey clearly shows that it did not preclude the use of various herbs and water as medicine. In addition to this, as we have already noted, repair and transplantation of various parts of the human body, including the head and limbs, find mention in the hymns, but based on current

[29] Krishnaswamy, *Āyurveda for the First-time Reader*, 12.

knowledge it is difficult to offer any scientific explanation for such allusions. At present, it can be noted that the scientific practice of surgical interventions referred to in the hymns cannot have been attained overnight. Such a body of knowledge suggests a long process of development in the traditional wisdom.

The Status of Physicians

According to the Vedic sources, a *bhiṣak* was a man of rituals. As is clear from the hymns, he was the custodian of the knowledge of healing rituals and the chanting of hymns as well as the qualities and potencies of herbs and the preparation of medicine. The treatment for diseases included the use of herbal medicines and the chanting of hymns.[30] Zysk compares this with the medicine men of South and North American Indians and their ritual dancing.[31] Quite significantly, a *bhiṣak* is described as a *prājña brāhmaṇa* (learned Brahmin), and more meaningfully a *vipra* (one who shakes) and a *mēdhāvi, rasavīryabhāvābhijño* (intelligent, one who knows the taste, quality, potency, the effect of transformation, and the curative power of herbs). The term *bheṣaja* is derived from *bhiṣak* and it refers to that which the healer uses in the curing rituals. On certain occasions, the term *bhiṣak* is used for referring to the gods. Thus, from the hymns we hear about Indra as a *bhiṣak* for sacrifice, Saraswati as a healing medicine, and Aśvinidevas as the divine healers. Significantly, *bhiṣak* appears along with a *takṣa*, carpenter, and a Brahmin, a priest, in a Rgvedic hymn that is dated to the late phase of the Vedic age.[32] Evidently, there was no restriction for others to practice medicine and this is apparent from the stories about the legendary physician Jīvaka.

Social differentiation and the *varṇa* (colour or caste) distinctions appear in a later phase of social formation. The earliest reference to the idea of *varṇa* suggesting a later social formation is in the hymn *Puruṣasūkta* in the tenth *maṇḍala* of the *Rgveda*. The *Taittiriyasamhita* makes a categorical statement: 'Therefore, medicine is not to be practised by a Brahmin for, he who is a physician, *bhiṣaj*, is impure, unfit

30 *Rgveda* 10, 97: 6.

31 Zysk, *Medicine in the Veda*, 7fn16.

32 *Rgveda* IX, 121: 1.

for the sacrifice.'[33] The *bhiṣak*, physicians, were considered inferior, especially when compared to the priestly section of the Vedic society. From an anthropological point of view, this is based on the idea of purity and pollution, which was shared by almost all primitive communities. According to sources, including the Brāhmaṇas and the *Dharmaśāstra*, they were not included in the sacrificial rites probably because they were considered impure and, therefore, polluting. The *Śatapatha Brāhmaṇa* makes a clear statement that the Aśvinidevas, the physicians of the celestial beings, were impure 'because they constantly roamed among the humans'.[34] The *Dharmaśāstra* texts, such as the laws of Manu, ordain that the food given by physicians must not be consumed, as it is like pus and blood.[35] This attitude has been explained from different angles. According to Debiprasad Chattopadhyaya, the root cause for the priestly contempt was a clash of philosophical perspectives between the basic empiricism of medical practice and the priestly ideology that emphasized esoteric knowledge.[36] Observing the whole problem from a sociological point of view, Kenneth Zysk maintains that the trend was there even in the earlier period probably due to their association with the *Atharvaveda*, which was not considered a principal text of the Ȩgvedic priests. Physicians frequently travelled to acquire knowledge regarding pharmacopoeia, which often brought them in contact with people outside the Vedic community. Such contact with sections of non-Aryan people must have given rise to an empirical orientation that became, as pointed out by Chattopadhyaya, antagonistic to the Brahminic orthodoxy in the later Vedic period.[37] Zysk adds in a convincing statement that the physicians earned their livelihood by administering cures and increased their knowledge by keen observation and also by exchanging clinical data they acquired from other physicians they came in contact with on

[33] Arthur B. Keith, *The Vedas of the Black Yajus School Entitled Taittiriya Sanhita*, 2 parts, Harward Oriental Series, nos. 18, 19 (Delhi: Motilal Banarsidass, 1967 [1914]), cviii.

[34] Jogiraj Basu, *India of the Age of the Brahmanas* (Calcutta: Sanskrit Pustaka Bhandar, 1969), 60.

[35] *Manusmṛti*, 3, 108: 152; 4, 212: 220. Reference is to the original text and not to any edited work.

[36] Debiprasad Chattopadhyaya, *The Science and Society in Ancient India* (Calcutta: Research India Publication, 1977), 212–14.

[37] Zysk, *Asceticism and Healing in Ancient India*, 224.

their travels. This contributed immensely to the development and growth of the science of Āyurveda at a later stage.[38]

The Epistemology of Vedic Healing

The mode of acquisition of the Vedic art of healing is, no doubt, magico-religious in nature, but at the same time it was also based on an objective knowledge of diseases and medicines. Thus, we hear about some kind of classification of diseases, such as *yakṣma* and *takman*, and this seems to imply some primary kind of reflexive thinking on the part of the practitioners of Vedic medicine during the period under consideration. This method of classification went on to become one of the several strategies used by scholars to understand a phenomenon. It is true that the origin of medicine was attributed to celestial beings in the form of myths and legends. At the same time, it has to be borne in mind that the purpose of the myths is not to provide information about the authorship of the knowledge. As we have noted earlier, this is done mainly to lend authority to a particular aspect.[39] Second, the legends on several occasions were aimed at appropriating valuable objects, including intellectual properties. The Vedic knowledge of diseases and medicines were accumulated over the course of several hundred years by many generations and such a fund of knowledge cannot claim authority based on its origin in a single fountainhead of knowledge and wisdom. Hence, the celestial beings appear as the originators of healing and healthcare.

Preservation and Transmission of Knowledge

Vedic hymns are *śrutis* in the sense that they are based on the sounds of the uttered word. This would suggest that they follow the principles of oral tradition. One of the characteristic features of oral traditions is the use of words, phrases, lines, and stanzas in the form of stock expressions. J. Gonda has shown how Vedic similes are composed by using the oft-repeated formulaic stock expressions.[40] Since the hymns

[38] Zysk, *Asceticism and Healing in Ancient India*, 20.

[39] Zysk, *Asceticism and Healing in Ancient India*, 213.

[40] J. Gonda, *Remarks on Similes in Sanskrit Literature* (Leiden: E.J. Brill, 1949), 22–3.

are oral in composition, they are transmitted orally by means of memorizing. Since the mantras are sacred, they should be free from errors and losses. A whole set of techniques of recitation of the entire corpus of hymns from beginning to end upwards and downwards, known as *jaṭa* and *ratha*, are in vogue even today among Vedic scholars. There are scholars, who can recite the whole body of the texts, thanks to these rigorous exercises.

The above features of the Vedic hymns seem to suggest that at an earlier stage of tribal social formation, the transmission of knowledge, including that of medicine, was in most cases within the *gotra* fraternity. However, this stage of social order had already given way to a stratified system of society by the time of the later Vedic *maṇḍalas*. Heterodox groups with their radical ideas of dissent and protest had already started appearing on the scene. In this new social setting, the transmission of the knowledge of the *bhiṣak*s in all probability was from father to son or in the absence of sons between members of the same family. At the same time, it has to be remembered that the exchange of ideas was common among different sections in the society such as tribal healers on the one hand and learned physicians on the other in the heterodox groups of Jains and Buddhists. Debates and discussions also took place among the different groups of experts in healing and healthcare. It may also be assumed that an empirico-rational idea of diseases and medicines was formed within the heterodox wandering healers, who did not believe in the Vedic or Brahminic pantheon and the magico-religious and ritual treatment.

A close look at the Vedic allusions to medicine and the art of healing would show that they belong to two distinctive stages in the development of the knowledge of medicine. The early phase is characterized by a primitive method of nature treatment—curing ailments by natural materials, such as water, heat, fire, and earth. The *Aithareya Brāhmaṇa* (1, 5: 2) states that fire or heat is the medicine to restore life. The *Śatapatha Brāhmaṇa* (5, 1: 4–6) states that 'within water is medicine'. The *Aithareya Brāhmaṇa* makes a noteworthy observation that rainwater charged with sun rays is a medicine or a potent drink. The Vedic seers had clear knowledge of toxicology and they knew that the remedy was sour things, such as tamarind, curd, and so on. The *Aithareya Brāhmaṇa* (2, 8: 4) reports a case of Mitra and Varuṇa who neutralized the intoxication by curd. This need not mean that herbal medicines were not known to the Vedic seers. There are some portions that regard Soma, the plant used in the *yajña* rituals, as the king of creepers and medicinal plants. The *Śatapatha Brāhmaṇa* (3, 1: 1–7) refers to an ointment for sores and itches.

It is possible from the foregoing account to delineate certain characteristic features of the knowledge of the Vedic medicine and the art of healing. First, the Vedic art of healing can be understood as belonging to two distinctive ages. The early stage, with the region being watered by the Indus river and its tributaries as its geographical background, was characterized by the practice of natural healing, that is, treatment by natural elements, and a large number of herbal medicines resulting from development in healthcare in a later phase. Second, the Vedic medicine was practised by the *bhiṣak*s with some amount of specialization. Their art of healing consisted of medicine supplemented by magical rites and the incantation of hymns. Third, the specialization of the *bhiṣak*s in the Vedic medical lore presupposes some amount of systematic organization of the knowledge of the science of a medicine accumulated during the long period from 1000 BCE to the middle of the first millennium BCE. Fourth, the medicinal knowledge of the *bhiṣak*s was supported and supplemented by auxiliary knowledge of the human anatomy, probably from experience in the sacrificial rituals. Fifth, there was a steady accumulation of knowledge about plants and plant life, including a vast amount of medicinal lore pertaining to the herbal plant. Sixth, and most significant, there was a parallel development of various traditions of rational thinking of the *Nyāya, Vaiśeṣika*, and the *Sānkhya* schools of philosophy. There was a trend of objective and rational explanations of diseases and their healing in the existing knowledge system. This was supported by the heterodox philosophical thinking of the Jains and the Buddhists, free from the hold of fear of Vedic deities and demons. This element of rational thinking was instrumental in bringing about a radical change, a paradigm shift, in the indigenous knowledge of the science of Āyurveda.

2

Towards Scientific Foundations of Healing

Buddhist Heterodox Tradition

The middle of the first millennium BCE was an age of tremendous changes in Indian history and culture. Social protest against Vedic ritualism and its inherent weaknesses was the force that was at work beneath these trends. Several ascetic teachers, such as Gautama Buddha, the Enlightened One; Makhali Gosāla of the Ājīvika sect; Nāthaputta of the Nirgrantha group; Mahāvīra of the Jains; and Pakuddha Kaccāyaṉa, the teacher of atomism, were working among the people, preaching their principles of heterodox ideas and ideals. Naturally, there were occasions when these teachers themselves entered into debates on conceptual problems. Romila Thapar observes that 'the thread of social protest winding through these heterodox teachings was indicative of a perception of change'.[1] According to Thapar, central to this awareness of change is the law of causality and 'it was

[1] Romila Thapar, 'Ethics, Religion and Social Protest', in her *Ancient Indian Social History* (Delhi: Oxford University Press, 1984), 50.

around this that much of the Buddhist doctrine revolves, claiming to derive from rational arguments and examples'.[2]

Causation of Diseases

The whole problem of the causes of diseases propounded by the Buddha has to be understood in the light of the world view of these philosophical systems (Figure 2.1). Buddhist canonical texts of the *Nikāyas* and the *Piṭakas* refer to some incidents in which the Buddha explains the causal connections of diseases. While talking with Gautama Buddha on the issue of the causes of the sufferings of mankind, a wandering monk Śivaka, evidently a physician appearing in the Jataka tales, said that according to some *śramaṇas* (Buddhist monks) and Brāhmaṇas, suffering was caused by karma, that is, previous acts only. Gautama Buddha replied that this view is incorrect. He explained that the cause of mankind's suffering was eightfold.[3]

(*i*) *pitta* (bile),
(*ii*) *sehma*[4] (phlegm),
(*iii*) *vāta* (wind), and
(*iv*) *sannipāta* (their combination)

are the primary causes. In addition to these, there are

(*i*) changes of the seasons,
(*ii*) stress of unusual activities,
(*iii*) going out hastily at night and being bitten by a snake, and
(*iv*) the result of action.

It is worth noting that this eightfold formula of the causation of diseases includes the three peccant humours. The close relation between these and the theory of *tridoṣa*, which is central to the science of Āyurveda, is unmistakable. Here, there is a question regarding the eighth cause, karma, as to whether it denotes *pūrvakarma*, the actions of the previous birth alone. According to the traditional Āyurvedic

[2] Thapar, 'Ethics, Religion and Social Protest', 51.

[3] *Samyuktanikāya*, 4: 230–1, *Anguttaranikāya*, 2: 87, and 3: 131. See also Zysk, *Asceticism and Healing in Ancient India*, 30.

[4] This is the Prakrit word. The Sanskrit form is *śleṣma*.

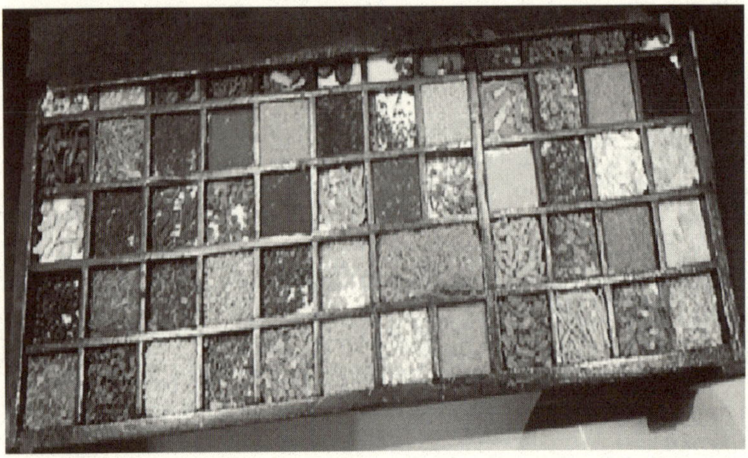

Figure 2.1 Medicine Box
Source: Author.

scholarship, karma could also signify the *āgantuka*, which is generally violent and traumatic and involves injury to the human body as in the case of judicial punishments and so forth.

The gradual development of the Buddhist monastic tradition of medicine, by the inclusion of rules pertaining to drugs and treatments for specific ailments rallied on codification of medical knowledge, is also present in a large part in the early Āyurvedic medical treatise. The congruence of these approaches strongly suggests a common origin for both the Buddhist monastery and the early Āyurvedic tradition. Legendary accounts and the Pāli texts show that the Buddhist monasteries played a significant role in the development of medical ethics.

The cultivation of land with effective iron tools and implements as indicated by archaeological evidences led to an unprecedented production of surplus. This prepared the ground for the development of trade and trading centres in the north and north-eastern regions of the Ganga–Yamuna valley as suggested by the urban archaeology of the period.[5] Famous towns such as Campa, Rājagṛha, Vaiśāli, Vārāṇasi, Kauśāmbi, Kuśinagara, Śrāvasti, and slightly later Pāṭalīputra rose to prominence during this period. Pāli texts mention as many as 20 towns

[5] R.S. Sharma, *Material Culture*, 16.

in the region. As we see in the literature, towns and markets were the places where artisans, craftsmen, and traders engaged in their activities. Historians underline the fact that the first lay converts to Buddhism were recruits from these traders.[6] The Buddhist teachings recommend some pattern of behaviour for the ideal trader and these are the qualities of an ideal monk too. More interestingly, monks are also advised to develop such qualities in them so they may understand the nature of *dukha*, worldly miseries, acquire proficiency in dharma, and take care of the monks who arrive from outside.[7]

The urban settings gave rise to certain features of city life. The urban surroundings and break-up of the old tribal system created a class of alienated women who took to prostitution as a source of livelihood. This was, to a certain extent, an encouragement for the pleasure-seeking interest of the wealthy section of society. Early Pāli literature relates how *gaṇikas*, public women, led a lofty life in the urban centres. Thus, Vaiśāli, a well-known city became famous due to its association with Amrapāli, a highly accomplished *gaṇika*. There are stories about how Bimbisāra, the king of Magadha and a contemporary of the Buddha, tried to bring a courtesan for his own city Rājagṛha. According to the Pāli texts, Buddhism maintained a soft attitude towards the Hindu *Dharmaśāstra*.

For a better understanding of the development, the period may be divided into two parts: The earlier one represented by the Buddhist Pāli canonical texts, and the later stage represented by the archaeology of the Buddhist monasteries and the epigraphic documents scattered therein over a vast area in the Deccan. Originally, the Buddha was preaching his new principles of life to the common people who gathered in important places for various purposes. Gradually, there was the necessity of the formation of congregations in the form of the Buddhist *saṅghas*. In the course of time, several people joined the *saṅgha* and it goes without saying that the members of such crowds needed some kind of healing practices. Quite naturally, the *bhikṣu*, mendicant saints, were closely in touch with the common people with their knowledge and wisdom, including their medicinal lore. The basic principle of the Buddhist religion was *karuṇa* (compassion) towards fellow beings and the major object of search was the strategy

6 Sharma, *Material Culture*, 124.

7 *Aṅguttara Nikāya*, 1, 117 (reference is to the original and not to any edited work).

to overcome worldly sufferings, and so it was their religious duty to develop some method for treating the different types of ailments of men and animals. Therefore, it is only logical to state that the Buddhist idea of medicine had in it a layer of folk-knowledge. Quite naturally, there were attempts at some level to suggest some causal connections between diseases and their causes.

It is not unlikely in the context of the materialist approach of the Buddhist principle that *kamma*, that is, the human acts in question, included the misdeeds and even crimes committed by the individuals. If this is acceptable, there were injuries too, among diseases, received by men from various sources, including judicial punishments for crimes committed by them. The *Dharmaśāstra* texts and the *Arthaśāstra* of Kautalya inform us that such punishments were awarded for criminal offences. There is every reason to believe that the services of surgeons were essential for the criminals to save themselves from danger and death. The *Suśrutasamhita* contains such a portion that describes the treatment of rhinoplasty in connection with the case of a nose that was cut off.[8]

The concept of the peccant humours, which is central to the Āyurvedic etiology, was most probably formulated in the Buddhist monasteries. The *Dīghanikāya* has an account of the human body in all its aspects and impurities. According to the description, in the body there is hair, nails, teeth, skin, flesh, sinuses, bones, bone marrow, kidney, heart, liver, pleura, spleen, lungs, bowels, intestines, stomach, excrements, bile, phlegm, semen, fat, tears, grease, saliva, mucous, serous fluid, and urine. The method suggests that anatomical knowledge was acquired originally by observing the parts of an animal as they were cut away from the body.[9] Another source of information was persistent attention on a decomposing corpse, thrown on a charnel ground.

Monastic Knowledge of Anatomy

The main source of the ascetic knowledge of the human anatomy was careful observation in the butcher houses. The *Dīghanikāya* prescribes that the monk should reflect on the body and learn its parts in the

[8] Varier, *History of Āyurveda*, 115; see also *Suśrutasamhita* 14: 46–50.

[9] Zysk, *Asceticism and Healing in Ancient India*, 34.

same way a skilled butcher or his skilful pupil does it.[10] Another way of collecting information about the human body involved the persistent observation of and concentrating on a decomposing corpse thrown on a charnel ground. The monk was also to reflect on a putrefying body dead for one to two days and being devoured by animals until its bones become bleached white and eventually turn to powder. It is this keen observation of decomposing bodies combined with the knowledge of the anatomy of animals gathered from the butcher's house that helped the early Buddhist monk-physicians to gather the basic information for understanding the gross internal and external structures of the human body. Being heterodox, the Buddhist were free from the Brahminical inhibitions regarding three kinds of practices: using *Atharvaveda*, touching outsiders for treatment, and travelling and associating with non-Brahminical sections.

Interestingly, at a later stage, the *Suśrutasamhita* has a separate section on another technique for obtaining knowledge of the human body involving a type of dissection:

> After having cleansed the corpse there is to be a complete visual ascertainment by the bearer of the knife [surgeon] who has a definite knowledge of the human body. One should learn what is visually perceived and what is taught in the text book. Then both together greatly increased one's understanding of the human body.[11]

The body should be cleaned after removing the faeces. It should not be badly injured and must not be too old (100 years old); the body must have a covering of *munja* grass, tree bark, *kusa* grass, or hemp, and so on. It should be placed in a cage or net and bound in a driving stream in a concealed spot. Then after seven nights the completely putrid body should be removed. One should very gradually scrape off successive layers of the body by means of *vetrivel* grass, coarse animal hair, or bamboo and should identify with the eyes all various major and minor parts of the body, both internal and external. This technique is not mentioned in the Pāli canons. However, accounts of travellers at a later date bear testimony to this practice even by Buddhists.

It may be noted in this connection that in the Western countries the early history of anatomy is shrouded in obscurity. Butchers had acquired some knowledge of animal anatomy from their profession.

[10] *Dīghanikāya* 2, 294: 22–6 and so forth.

[11] Zysk, *Asceticism and Healing in Ancient India*, 35.

Scholars have observed that the ancient Greeks pursued animal anatomy, and that in the beginning of that knowledge anatomy was only animal anatomy except in the school of Alexandria in the third century BCE.[12] The rediscovery of the fine structure of the body and codification of the essential knowledge of human anatomy was an achievement of the Renaissance. According to some textbooks on surgery, the first manual for dissection was written by Mondino de Luzzi in 1316.[13] It was only in the mid-fifteenth century that a special theatre was established at Padna for anatomic dissection.

An empirical knowledge of human anatomy on the basis of dissection and direct observation of human body is fundamental to Āyurvedic medical science. In all probability this can be understood as an influence of the Buddhist tradition. Kenneth Zysk observes that a vast storehouse of medical knowledge developed among the *sramana* physicians supplies the Indian medical tradition with the precepts and practices of what comes to be known as Āyurveda. The first documented codification of this medical lore took place as wandering ascetics assumed a more stationary existence cloistered in the early Buddhist monastery.[14]

In Greek and the Roman antiquity, physicians turned to surgery only when drugs were not available. Hippocrates figures prominently in the history of Greek works though all works were not written by a single individual. One of such works is entitled *On the Surgery*. The author says that surgeons should know how they should proceed with treatment. Much of the work pertains to the work of bandaging various types of injuries. Hippocrates wrote around 400 BCE that the things related to surgery are the patient, the operator, the assistants, the instruments, the light, the where and how, the how many things and how, the time, the manner, and the place.[15]

By the thirteenth and fourteenth centuries, surgery was denigrated and avoided by physicians who had received their education in the universities that were rising all over Europe. Medicine was usually one of the basic subjects of study. Surgeons, on the other hand, very

[12] Girt H. Brieger, 'The Development of Surgery', in *Text Book of Surgery: The Biological Basis of Modern Surgical Practice*, Vol. I, ed. David C. Sabiston (Bangalore: Saunders, 1994), 1–4.

[13] Varier, *History of Āyurveda*, Chapters 19, 20.

[14] Zysk, *Asceticism and Healing in Ancient* India, 37.

[15] Varier, *History of Āyurveda*.

often came from the unlettered lower classes and they were scorned in clerical circles. According to the available sources, the surgeons were taught the ways of their craft by apprenticeship.[16]

The regular and systematic fund of medical knowledge was developed in the Buddhist monastic institutions as the ascetic physicians travelled from place to place treating sick monks, lay devotees, and also the common people. Systematic pedagogical programmes and methods of treatment were also developed most probably in Buddhist monasteries. Takṣasila (Taxila), often described as an ancient university, was perhaps the most renowned among the high seats of learning for various disciplines, including the science of Āyurveda. Famous physicians like the semi-legendary Ātreya were teachers of Takṣasila, while Jīvaka Komarabhacha was a product of Takṣasila. He studied for seven years as a disciple of the physician Atreya whose teachings formed the basis of the *Carakasamhita*.

Knowledge of Medicine

The earliest codification of medical knowledge in India is perhaps in the Buddhist canonical work *Mahāvagga* attributed with the authority of Gautama Buddha himself as in the case of the monastic code as a whole. It is difficult to examine whether all the cases featured in the work were on the basis of consultations with the Buddha. However, what is important is that when compared with the later Samhitas of Caraka, Suśruta, and Bheḷa many similarities can be found between the two traditions while at the same time there are differences too. The monastic medicine is generally taken to represent an early attempt to provide a manual of medical practices and perhaps that is why the authority was registered with the Enlightened One. Most probably it was for claiming legitimacy for the practices and in all probability, this was the source of the formalized collections detailed in the later Buddhist medical recipe books, such as the portion *Nāvanītaka* contained in the Bower manuscript, Nāgārjuna's *Yōgaśataka*, Ravigupta's *Siddhasāra*, and the *Jīvaka Pustakam*.

As explained in the Buddhist texts, basic medicines were prescribed by the Buddha for different ailments. They are fats, roots, extracts, leaves, fruits, gums or resins, and salts. Fat consisted of those

16 Brieger, 'The Development of Surgery', 1–4.

drawn from bears, fish, swine, donkey, and so forth. Later, Buddhaghōṣa too elaborates on fats as medicine. He says that fat from the flesh of all edible animals and of the 10 inedible animals can be used as medicine. Buddhaghōṣa advises that the oil made from the fats is to be used as medicine. The permitted roots were turmeric, ginger, sweet flag, Indian atees, black hellebore, vettiver, and nut grass. This can be compared with Caraka who enumerates 16 plants that have useful roots, none of which occurres in the list of the Pāli texts. Extracts or *kaṣāya* were needed by the monks. Buddha allowed the extracts from the following: neem tree, *kuṭaja* tree, *pakkava* tree, and Indian beech. It may be noted in this connection that Caraka explains 50 extracts. Monks required leaves to be used as medicine. The Buddha permitted the following: neem, *kuṭaja*, *paṭola*, holy basil, and *kārpāsika* (cotton tree). Fruits were also used as medicine by the monks with the permission of Buddha himself. These consisted of *viḍaṅga*, long pepper, black pepper, yellow *myrobalan*, *emblic myrobalan*, and so forth. Any fruit that does not serve as solid or soft food was allowed by the Buddha to be used as medicine. The classification of fruits as a separate category of medicinal fruits is common to both the Buddhist monastic medicine and the early Āyurvedic medicine. Sikh monks required gums or resins (*jatu*) as medicine. Resins from asafoetida were allowed by the Buddha. Here Buddhaghoṣa explains that asafoetida had three other varieties. According to him, there are other resins or lac (*lākṣa*), such as *sarjarasa*. Jatu or *sasarja* (a mineral used in Āyurveda) is rarely used in the medical treatises, such as the *Suśrutasamhita*. Interestingly, a group of drugs under the category of resins developed in the tradition of Suśruta is not found in other extant medical traditions. Monks required salts as medicine. Buddha permitted the following ones: (*a*) ocean salt, (*b*) black salt, (*c*) rock salt, and (*d*) red salt. A close parallel can be found in Caraka who enumerates five salts very similar to the Pāli tradition. Suśruta treats them individually and adds to the list three more basic salts such as *guḍika*, *kuṭa*, and *kṣāra*.

Monastery and Medicine

The interest in medicine had different dimensions. It was in a way related to yogic practices. Romila Thapar observes that the Buddhist Nāgārjuna summed it up when he referred to the transformation of *prakṛti* (substance) by the use of *oṣadhi* and *samādhi* (meditation). Thapar observes that it is not surprising that the earliest compendia of medicine, that of Suśruta, is associated with Nāgārjuna.

> 'Equally interesting and logical is the fact that Taxila, apart from being a culturally cosmopolitan town, was renowned as a high seat of medical knowledge with important Buddhist monasteries. Megasthenes, in his discriptions of the *śramaṇas*, states that some form of approximate medicine was practised by the ascetic sects. In the Buddhist and the Jaina tradition attending to the medical well being of the lay community is incumbent upon the monk.'[17]

Medical knowledge was not unfamiliar to the ascetic wanderers from the sixth century BCE. It has been considered that especially during the days of Buddhism it was part of the religious doctrines and the monastic discipline. *Mahāvagga* (8: 26) relates how the Buddha's own experience led to the realization that the monks should help themselves since there was nobody to take care of them. Once, the Buddha was going on a round of inspection, visiting monks in their cells. He found a monk who was sick and was suffering from dysentery. The monk had fallen from his bed and he was lying in his own ordure. Buddha washed the sick man with his own hands and laid him comfortably on his bed.

This signalled the starting of a new rule to the order. The Buddha told the monks: 'Brethren, you have no mother or father to care for you. If you do not care for one another who else will do so?' A.L. Basham suggests that it was under the influence of such teachings that Ashoka established free hospitals, and that Buddhist monks have at all times studied medical lore, and treated laymen as well as their own fellows.[18]

The use of food as medicine is extremely interesting not only from the angle that it saw a steady relaxation of the monastic rules but also in that it sheds much welcome light on the amazing knowledge that the Buddhists possessed on various medicinal herbs and surgical operations. An incomplete but fairly impressive list of these articles include sandalwood, chunam, various kinds of gums, salt, leaves, fruits, and stringent decoctions. The *Mahāvagga* indicates that they

[17] Romila Thapar, 'Renunciation; A Counter-culture?', in her *Ancient Indian Social History* (Hyderabad: Orient Longman, 1984), 96.

[18] Basham, *Wonder That Was India*, 285.

were aware of surgical therapy and they performed it.[19] This is a pointer to the contribution of these monasteries to the knowledge and practice of Indian medicine.

The Buddhist monasteries in the period under consideration served as resting places for caravans where they had food, lodging, and medicine for the sick. Most of the monasteries were situated on the trade routes and near the towns, which were the centres of activities of mercantile communities. This is of great significance in analysing their mutual relationship.

Animal urine (usually from cattle) is included in the medical section of the *Vinaya* as the allowable treatment for snake bites.[20] It is mentioned in the *Mahāvagga* and in the early Āyurvedic treatises as a principle ingredient in a number of recipes and therapies.[21] Medicines included all those things necessary for the care of the sick and were to be used only to ward off pain and to maintain health, never to give pleasure (*Sabbasava Sutta*, 27/*Majjhima nikāya* 1, 1: 10). The chapter on medicines (*bhasajia khandhaka*) of the *Mahāvagga* specifies the requisite medicines. The five basic medicines: clarified butter (ghee or *sappi*, Skt *srpis*), butter (*navanīta*), oil (*taila*), honey (*madhu*), and molasses (*phanita*) were permitted for the monks. With the evolution of the *saṅgha* and the development of the *vinaya* rules, the medicine grew into an entire pharmacopoeia, including numerous items of food. Early Buddhist texts, including the *Mahāvagga*, inform us that the early monastic establishment provided store rooms for food stuffs (*kappiyabhūmi*) and persons such as *khajjabhajaka*s (who distribute solid food), *yavāgubhajaka*s (who distribute gruel), and *phalabhajaka*s (who distribute fruits).[22]

Management of Diseases

The development of the materia medica in the Buddhist *saṅgha* seems to have taken place on the basis of a systematic classification of foods.

19 *Mahāvagga* 6, 22: 4. Reference is to the original text and not to any edited text.

20 *Mahāvagga* 6, 14: 6.

21 *Carakasamhita*, *Sūtrasthāna* 1, 69–14: 4, *Cikitsitasthāna* 10, 41; *Suśruta*, 15, 5: 11. 45, 217: 26.

22 *Mahāvagga*, 1, 30: 40; 6, 17: 1–6.

The early Āyurvedic treatises also contain a similar system of the classification of foods. There was a gradual transition from the restricted medical care of monks of the fellow *bhikṣus* to the institutionalized mechanism in the *saṅgha*, as the situation demanded. The *Mahāvagga* identifies the qualities (*aṅga*) of easy and difficult patients and of competent and incompetent nurses. The comparison of these regulations with the qualities of *sadhya* and *asādhya paricārakas* (competent and incompetent nurses) given in the classical Āyurvedic texts sheds much light on the evolution of the science. Though the quality of physician, patient, medical attendant, and medicine prescribed in the early medical treatises are not identical with those found in the *Vinayapiṭaka*, they share many points in common. It may also be noted that Caraka's standardization of the four qualities appears to be closer to the lists contained in the Buddhist tradition. It may be added in this connection, as observed by some recent scholars, that medical care in the monastic centres and the early medical treatment in Āyurveda strongly suggest continuities in medical doctrine and practice. It has also been opined that both the systems were derived from a common source of medical lore.[23]

The most renowned physician of the Jātaka tales is Jīvaka Komārabhacca. The *Mahāvagga* mentions a famous physician Jīvaka, with an epithet Komārabhacca. A contemporary of Gautama Buddha, he is mentioned as providing free medical care to Buddha and other monks. There are several stories in the Jātaka tales and in the Tibetan songs about this physician and his treatment. Commenting on the description of Suśruta, Ḍalhaṇa includes the name of Jīvaka in the list of the masters of *kaumārabhṛtya* (paediatrics).[24] It appears that the early source of the Jīvaka legends must be the Buddhist texts, including the *Nikayas* and the *Pitakas*. The *Mahāvagga* relates the story of Jīvaka: Śālāvati, a courtesan of Rajgir, discarded her newborn baby in a dustbin. Prince Abhaya saved the baby and brought him up in the palace. As life was restored to him after being discarded, he was named Jīvaka; also, he was called Komārabhacca for being reared by the prince (Kumāra). After formal education, he went to Taxila with the blessings of the king and studied medicine for seven years. Having passed all the tests prescribed, he returned home. On his way

[23] Zysk, *Asceticism and Healing in Ancient India*, 37, 86.
[24] Sharma, *Caraka Samhita*.

back, he cured the chronic headache of a merchant's wife in Magadha by nasal drops. The couple offered him a chariot, some retinues, and enormous wealth. He wished to offer everything to the prince who was his benefactor, but the prince returned all of them to Jīvaka. Later, he cured Bimbisāra, the king of Magadha, from fistula by applying an ointment; pleased with the treatment, the king offered Jīvaka 500 gaily-decked ladies and entrusted him with the treatment of the Buddhist monks residing in his court. He miraculously cured the chronic headache of a merchant; Jīvaka made the patient unconscious, opened his skull and removed two worms that caused the suffering. He relieved a patient of Benaras who was suffering from hernia through a surgery of the abdomen, and was amply rewarded. He treated Pradyota, the king of Ujjain, for leukoderma; as the king refused to take the medicated ghee, Jīvaka gave it in the form of a decoction. On consuming it, the king vomited; knowing that the king was short-tempered, he escaped and returned to Rajagraha. The king got cured of his ailment and sent many presents to Jīvaka. Jīvaka restored Buddha's health by means of purgation (*virecana*). Jīvaka offered all the presents he received to the Buddha for the use of monks.

Another story, according to Tibetan songs, goes like this: A boy, born to Bimbisāra in Bhujiṣya, was discarded in a basket. The boy was saved and brought up by Prince Abhaya and hence got the name Kumārabhṛta/Kaumārabhṛtya. He studied medicine and was sent to Taxila for specialization in surgery of the head. He got trained under Atreya and attained such proficiency that he surpassed even his *ācārya*.

Jīvaka in the *Kāśyapasamhita*

Jīvaka of *Kāśyapasamhita* is not connected with the above stories. He was not a resident of Rājagṛha nor was he a son of Bimbisāra, begotten by a courtesan. He hailed from Kaṉakhala and he was the son of sage Ècīka. As the story goes, he became grey and shrunken at the age of five and came to be called 'aged Jīvaka'. He was the disciple of Kāśyapa (the keeper of agni [fire]), not of Atreya. Jīvaka was the master of the Vedas, a devotee of jīvakāśyapa (founder of the clan), and the ancestor of Vātsya who redacted the *Kāśyapasamhita*. He was a follower of the *Śrutis* (vedas) and the *Smṛtis* and not a Buddhist. Jīvaka, the contemporary of Buddha, as is evident from the stories related to him, was mainly a surgeon. But Jīvaka, the compiler of the *Kāśyapasamhita*, was the author of the work on *kaumārabhṛtya*.

Buddhist stories show the contemporaneity of Kāśyapa and Jīvaka but they are not the Kāśyapa and Jīvaka mentioned in the *Kāśyapasamhita*. The *Mahāvagga* describes Kāśyapa of the Buddhist stories but there are no indications that this Kāśyapa was a physician, paediatrician, or master of *tantras* rather than a philosopher; nor is he the son of Marīci. According to the Tibetan songs, Jīvaka studied at Taxila under Atreya but Jīvaka in the Samhita was a disciple of Kāśyapa of Magadha. Thus, the Buddhist Kāśyapa and the Kāśyapa of the Samhita tradition are different. Jīvaka of the Buddhist stories was brought up by Kumāra and that was how he became Komārabhacca in the Pāli language, whereas the *Kāśyapasamhita* says that Jīvaka became Kaumārabhṛtya because he was the author of the work on paediatrics (*kaumārabhṛtya*). The term *kaumārabhṛtya* can be seen extensively used for paediatrics in Suśruta and Nāvanītaka. Jīvaka of the *Kāśyapasamhita* was never a Buddhist, nor does his work show any Buddhist trend; surgery was mentioned in his text only casually.

Jīvaka in the Jaina Works

Some Jaina works contain the story of Jīvaka. But this Jīvaka had many aliases, such as prince Śrutandhara, Jīvandhara, Jīvasvami, and so forth. Some of the Jaina works relate the story of this Jīvaka. However, he does not seem to be credited with the status of an *ācārya* of medicine or proficient in pediatrics. Moreover, the Buddhist or the Jaina traditions are absent in the *Kāśyapasamhita*; it goes back to the true Vedic tradition.

The texts mention only the attendant or nurse who functions along with the healer. Legends and stories relate how lay women also provided medical services to both monks as well as nuns. Suppiya, a lay devotee, was the best example, known for her services for sick monks and nuns.[25] She was famous as a nurse to the *saṅgha*. According to a legend in the same text, she undertook an extreme act of piety, a piece of flesh from her own body to be used in the broth for a sick man in the absence of

25 I.B. Horner, *Women under Primitive Buddhism: Laywomen and Almswomen* (Delhi: Motilal Banarsidass, 1930), 333–4.

meat (Mahāvagga 6, 23: 1–3; *Amguttaranikāya* 1, 14: 7). A physician named Ākāsagotta of Rājagaha allegedly lanced a rectal fistula, which was a forbidden act for monks to perform.

State and Medicine: The Mauryan Period

Buddhist monasteries and their medicinal services were probably instrumental in spreading the knowledge and practice of medicine to a vast area in and outside the regions of the subcontinent. We hear for the first time about this cultural expansion from the Mauryan sources. The major Girnar Edict II of the Mauryan emperor Ashoka speaks about this historical event:

> Everywhere in the dominions of King Devānāmpriya priyadarśi and likewise among his borders such as the Cholas, Pandyas, Sathyaputhras, Keralaputhras even Tāmraparni, the Yavana king Antiyaka, and also kings who are the neighbours of this Antiyaka – everywhere, two kinds of medical treatments – that is, for humans and for cattles – are established by king Devānāmpriya priyadarśi. Wherever the herbs that are beneficial to humans and cattles are not available, they are brought and planted. Wherever there were no fruits and roots they are brought and planted. Wells were caused to be dug, trees were caused to be planted on routes for the use of men and cattles.[26]

This royal proclamation is supported by excavated materials from different parts of the subcontinent and also from beyond the borders, such as Sri Lanka, to show that the science of Āyurveda was spread outside its original places of origin and developments during the Mauryan period (see, for example, Figure 2.2). Historical relics from Tissarama, a site in Ceylon, may be taken as the best example. The excavation materials at Tissamaharama include, according to the studies, relics of old buildings with clay floors and a large number of saddles and querns for preparing herbal medicines including *lehyas* (medicines that are consumed by licking), pastes, and *gulikas* (pills) as prescribed in the Āyurvedic pharmacopoeia. It is interesting to note in this connection

[26] E. Hutzsch, *Corpus Inscriptionum Indicarum*, Vol. I: Inscriptions of Asoka (Delhi: Archaeological Survey of India, 1991 [1922], 2–4).

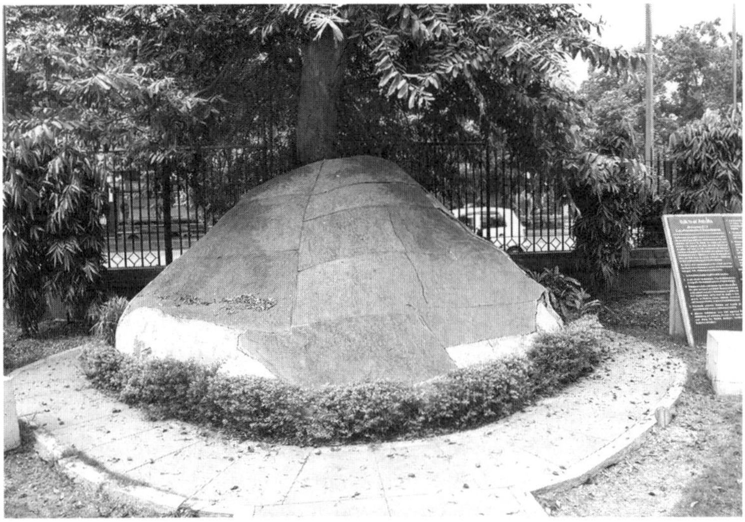

Figure 2.2 Girnar Edict II
Source: Author.

that *Mahavamśa*, the historical chronicle of Ceylon, refer to a centre of health at this place.[27]

In the post-Mauryan period, there are several Brahmi label inscriptions at Buddhist sites in Maharashtra and Deccan regions, such as Karle, Kanheri, Kuda, Pitalkhora, and so forth. These epigraphic documents from North India as well as South India are replete with references to various aspects of therapeutic strategies and the functionaries who were involved in such activities. Inscriptional references to the centres for healthcare are brought out from various places in the subcontinent. The structural remains of a building with four rooms of varying sizes were excavated at Kumrahār, the ancient Mauryan capital Pāṭalīputra. This came from the layer representing the period from 300 to 450 CE. It is learnt from the excavation reports of Kumrahar that the structures consisted of a building with four

[27] Heidrun Schenk and Hans-Joachim Weissharr, 'The Citadel of Tissamaharama: Urban Habitat and Commercial Interrelations', in *Ports of the Ancient Indian Ocean*, ed. Marie Francoise Boussac, Jean Francoise Sallers, and Jean Baptiste (Delhi: Primus, 2016).

rooms in different sizes.[28] The excavated materials include a seal with an inscription in the Gupta Brahmi characters, which reads 'Srī āryogyavihāre bhikṣusaṅghasya' (monastery of the Buddhist monks). This reminds us of the *ārōgya vihāras* (hospitals) of the Buddhist literature. Two potsherds were also obtained from the same site with labels written in the same script 'Ārogyavihāre Dhanvantare', meaning Dhanwanthari's centre of healthcare. The paleographic features of the inscription help to date the artefact to the Gupta age, that is, from the fourth century CE. It may also be remembered along with this that according to widely popular legends, Dhanwanthari was one among the *navaratna*, nine gems, that adorned the royal court of Chandragupta Vikramāditya, the Gupta emperor and celebrated hero of numerous legends. The other gems of the royal court were Kṣapaṇaka, a Jaina mathematician; Amarasimha, the classical lexicographer; Śanku (whose identity is doubtful); Vetāḷa-bhatta, a faithful bodyguard of the king; Ghaṭakarpara and Kāḷidāsa, two well-known poets; Varahamihira, the astronomer and the author of *Bṛhadsamhita*, an encyclopaedic volume on astronomy; and Vararuchi, also an astronomer. An inscription yielded by a monastic site at Konda in Andhra Pradesh reads 'vihāramukhye vigatajvarālaye' (monastery meant for those who have been cured of their illness). These archaeological remains clearly inform us that arrangements for the establishment of systematic treatment for in-patients were made by authorities in places where there was a demand for the same.

The accounts of the Chinese traveller Fa-Hsien records that the heads of some Vaiśya[29] families in the city of Pāṭalīputra established houses for dispensing medicines to the poor, the destitute, and the handicapped. We learn from these accounts that there were physicians who would attend the patients and provide the necessary treatment for the patients in such homes. The patients were provided food and medicine.[30] It may be remembered along with this that tools and instruments such as mortars and pestles were excavated from the sites of monasteries at Sāranāth, from the layers belonging to the

[28] A. S. Altekar and Vijayakanta Misra, *Report on Kumrahar Excavations, 1951–1955* (Patna: K.P. Jayaswal Research Institute, 1959). See also Romila Thapar, *From Lineage to State* (Bombay: OUP, 1984), 71.

[29] The third *varṇa*, the others being Brahmin, Kṣatriya, and Śūdra.

[30] James Legge, *The Travels of Fâ-hien* (reprint) (New Delhi: Master Publishers, 1981), 79.

ninth century CE.[31] These tools and implements are taken by scholars to indicate that monasteries were preparing Āyurvedic medicines, such as *cūrṇa* (powder), *kaṣāya*, and so forth for providing preparations, nursing, and treatment for the patients. A copper-plate inscription from the south-eastern part of Bengal dated 930 CE, edited and published by D.C. Sircar, informs us that King Srīcandra made arrangements for providing one physician for each of the two *maṭhas* (residences).[32]

Material Milieu of Monastic Centres in the Deccan

Kautalya refers to the rich resources of minerals along the *dakṣināpatha*, the southern route, connecting the Ganga valley with the regions beyond the Vindhyan ranges. He extols the advantages of the land route over sea routes. In the western Deccan, there is a notable transformation during the rise of the Sātavāhanas, which is characterized by a proliferation of urban centres and a parallel increase in the Buddhist monastic establishments.[33] Trade, both internal and external, increased during this period resulting in an increase in the number of traders and their paraphernalia who depended on these institutions for rest, protection, and support. Itinerary monks, including those with knowledge of medicine, must have been visiting these institutions for various purposes.

[31] Deepak Kumar Barua, *Viharas in Ancient India: A Survey of Buddhist Monasteries* (Calcutta: Indian Publications, 1969), 120.

[32] D.C. Sircar, *Epigraphic Discoveries in East Pakistan* (Calcutta: Sanskrit College, 1973), 35.

[33] Himanshu P. Ray, *Monastery and Guild* (Delhi: OUP, 1986), 110–12. See also *Maharashtra State Gazetteer* (Maharashtra: Government of Maharashtra, 1975), 517–18.

3

The Age of the Samhitas

The science of Āyurveda attained maturity in the classical texts of the Samhitas. There are several Samhitas and each of them is attached to the name of an *ācārya*, preceptor, such as Caraka, Suśruta, Bhēḷa, Kāśyapa, Hārīta, and so forth. Better knowledge and wisdom of indigenous healing and healthcare is explained in the Samhitas with special references to a particular branch of the science. Thus, *kāyacikitsa*, general medicine, is the subject of the *Carakasamhita*, while surgery is the subject of the *Suśrutasamhita*. Bhēḷa deals with the mind, Kāśyapa focuses on pediatrics, while Hārīta deals with a variety of topics such as *dravyaguṇa*, property of herbs and other medicinal objects; *riṣṭalakṣaṇa*, signs of death; systems of measurements; and the like. What is preserved in the preceding literature, including the Vedas, the Brāhmaṇas, and the Buddhist Pāli canonical texts, as seeds and seedlings of healing and healthcare is found fully grown in the Samhitas nourished by scholarly discussions and analytical thought at various levels. The ancient Indian system of medicine was designated as Āyurveda by the time of the Samhitas.

The questions of authorship and authority of transmission of the knowledge of Āyurveda appear for the first time in the Samhitas. The origin of Āyurveda is attributed to celestial beings, such as Indra, Brahma, and so on, thereby claiming a divine origin of the knowledge. The *ācāryas* of the Samhitas remain silent about the monastic tradition and its contributions to the development and growth of the science of Āyurveda.

Caraka's Version

According to Caraka, Indra revealed the science to Bharadvāja. Towards the end of *Kṛtayuga*, 'the Golden Age', justice waned and selfish people began to accumulate more wealth. Gradually, they fell prey to evil passions and subsequently to diseases. Diseases took away long life from them. The sages pitied them and they assembled on the slopes of the Himalayas to find a remedy for human suffering. In this connection, a special reference is made to sages such as Angiras and many others. They sent Bharadvāja to Indra to learn Āyurveda. Indra was pleased with him and revealed to him the secrets of medicines. From Bharadvāja it passed on through Ātreya to Agniveśa, Bheḷa, Jatukarṇa, Parāśara, Hārīta, and Kṣārapāṇi. These sages compiled their own Samhitas.

Suśruta's Version

Suśruta states that Āyurveda is auxiliary to the *Atharvaveda*. Brahma created it even before he created human beings. According to Suśruta, Prajāpati learned it from Brahma, the twin gods Aśvinidevas from Prajāpati, Indra from the Aśvinidevas, and Divodāsa from Indra. Divodāsa is another name for Dhanvantari. From Dhanvantari a group of disciples, including Suśruta, Aupadhenava, Vaitaraṇa, Aurabhra, Puṣkalāvata, Kara, Vīrya (or Karavīrya), Gopurarakṣita, Nimi, Bhoja, Kaṅkāyana, Gālava, and Garga, learnt the science with emphasis on surgery and compiled their own texts. All of the Samhitas endorse the lineage up to Indra.

Kāśyapa's Version

According to Kāśyapa, Vasiṣṭha, Atri, and Bhṛgu learnt it from Indra. They passed it on to their sons and disciples. Jīvaka compiled *Kāśyapasamhita*. Jīvaka, Parvataka, and Bandhuka composed paediatric treatises. The sages received from Indra the Āyurveda with all its eight branches. Divodāsa laid stress on surgery, Ātreya on medicine, and Kāśyapa on paediatrics.

Aṣṭāṅgahṛdaya

Vāgbhaṭa follows Caraka and Suśruta and explains that Brahma recalled and revealed it, thereby signifying that creation is only the revelation of what has already been in existence. Actually, Brahma remembered it, thereby implying that the knowledge had been in existence and hence he could remember the same. Brahma revealed it to Prajāpati. He passed it over to Indra, Ātreya, and others.

Legend in the Purāṇas

The stories in the Puranic sources are different from the versions found in the Samhitas. An example is the *Brahmavaivarta purāṇa*. According to this, Prajāpati elevated Āyurveda like the four Vedas and revealed it to the Sun, who compiled the Samhita and presented it to his 16 disciples. Each of them composed their own Samhitas.

Āyurveda also prescribes treatments for animals, birds, and plants. The sage Sālihōtra composed Aśvāyurveda for horses and Mātaṅga composed Hastyāyurveda for elephants. Āyurveda for trees (Vṛkṣāyurveda) was composed by Surapāla but all these are subdivisions of Brahma's Āyurveda. According to the *Agnipurāṇa*, Dhanvantari imparted to Suśruta the Āyurveda for man, elephant, horse, cattle, and trees.

It may be noted that there is no uniformity among the Samhitas about the pedigree through which knowledge was transmitted. At the same time, it has to be borne in mind while discussing this aspect that a huge fund of knowledge as that of Āyurveda is generally not invented or formulated by a single individual. It is accumulated in course of time, thanks to the big and small contributions of numerous individuals as well as groups and persons. Against this idea, the various origin myths acquire new meaning and significance.

It is clear from Table 3.1 that most of the legendary accounts trace the origin of Āyurveda either to Indra or to Brahma and consider it as a part of the Vedic lore. But alchemy, which is a prominent part of Āyurveda, owes its allegiance to the Śaiva tradition (the tradition related to the faith of Śiva). Āyurveda in its original form was vast, and

Table 3.1 The Lineage of *Ācāryas* and Their Preceptors

Brahma			
Prajāpati			
Aśvinidevas			
Indra			
According to the *Carakasamhita*	According to the *Suśrutasamhita*	According to the *Kāśyapasamhita*	According to the *Aṣṭāṅgahṛdaya* and *Aṣṭāṅgasaṅgraha*
Indra	Indra	Indra	Indra
Bharadvāja	Divodāsa (Dhanvantari)	Vasiṣṭha, Athri, Bhrugu	Ātreya
Ātreya Agniveśa Bheḷa Jatukarṇa Parāśara Hārīta Kṣārapāṇi	Suśruta	Jīvaka	

Source: Varier, *History of Āyurveda*, 112.

varied in content. It is said that there were 1,00,000 verses and 1,000 chapters in Brahma's Āyurveda. But the Samhitas and *tantras* available today have only 120 chapters in 8 parts. They were abridged to the present form due to the short span of human life and also due to the limited power of intelligence of the people of later ages! In the *Kṛtayuga*[1], men lived for 400 years. In the succeeding ages, the lifespan became shorter and shorter. In *Kaliyuga*, this came down to a mere 120 years. So, for the benefit of those who were not as intelligent as those in the olden days, it was necessary to abridge the Āyurveda so as to enable men to learn it in their short lifespan.

Origin myths are approached from different angles. It has been maintained by scholars of cultural anthropology, such as B. Malinowski, that myths are essentially charters of validation in which the aim was very often to provide sanction for current situations. According to them, myths made the past intelligible and meaningful.[2] Following Malinowski, Romila Thapar maintains that myths from earlier periods

[1] One among the four yugas. The others are Tretayuga, Dwāparayuga, and Kaliyuga.

[2] B. Malinowski, *Magic, Science and Religion* (New York: Orient Longman, 1948) quoted in Thapar, *Ancient Indian Social History*.

are recast in conformity with the social assumptions of later periods.[3] The repetition of the same myths with, perhaps, some modification, from age to age is partly to ensure the message getting through and partly to indicate new nuances. Myths are also understood as archetypes and as a primary cultural force. Romila Thapar suggests that they are generally used not for recording any historical truth but to claim some kind of legitimacy for something.[4] Against this intellectual background, it becomes somewhat clear why the Indra myth eclipsed and appropriated the contributions of the heterodox sections of the Jaina and the Buddhist preceptors while tracing the story of the development of the science of Āyurveda. Similarly, we need not be misled by the Brahma myth that projects a later Brahminical view, which is in all probability an attempt at claiming and appropriating the authorship of the invaluable tradition of the science of health by later Brahminic sections.

Caraka

Caraka is associated with the redaction of the work of the great physician Agniveśa who compiled the teachings of the great *ācārya*, Ātreya. Rudra, the commentator of *Bṛhajjātaka*, introduces Caraka as a scholar of Āyurveda and as a *bhikṣu* wandering for the well-being of mankind. The term *caraka* denotes different meanings on different occasions. Referring to *Bhāvaprakāśa*, modern scholars, such as N.V.K Varier, are of the view that Ananta, a master of all the six *Vedaṅgas* and Āyurveda, wandered all over the world in the guise of a sage to learn about worldly life.[5] The term *caraka* is taken to be derived from this habit of wandering. It is not unlikely that Caraka, the redactor of the Āyurvedic text, belonged to the clan of the wandering *carakas*.

Caraka redacted the *Agniveśatantra*. Redaction is the process in which the author expands the condensed aphorisms to make them more explicit and also summarizes elaborate statements of the original wherever necessary; this gives a new form to the original

[3] Romila Thapar, 'Origin Myths and the Early Indian Historical Tradition', in her *Ancient Indian Social History* (Hyderabad: Orient Longman, 1984), 297.

[4] Thapar, 'Origin Myths', 297.

[5] Varier, *History of Āyurveda*, 90.

work. Thus, the verses added during the discussion and also at the end of the chapters are by the redactor or the redactors. *Carakasamhita* in its complete form was not available due to mutilation and so forth during the time of Dṛḍhabala. He worked upon the remains of the lost and mutilated portions. The 13th chapter of the *Sūtrasthāna* enumerates the names of all the chapters. Based on this, he filled up the missing portions; the portions in verses are ascribed to him and whatever can be seen in prose is the restored portion from the mutilated parts of the *Carakasamhita*. On the basis of external and internal evidences, Caraka is assigned by some scholars to the first century CE, the flourishing period of the Mahāyāna movement in Buddhism, and the great physician is believed to be a scholar who adorned the royal court of the Kuṣana king Kaniṣka.

Carakasamhita

The *Carakasamhita* is the basic work available today on the science of medicine. The treatise gets its name from the author Caraka but the identity and dates of the author are subjects of unending controversy. Each of the chapters of the treatise ends with a note on its compilation: 'made by Agniveśa, redacted by Caraka and updated by Dṛḍhabala'. Dṛḍhabala updated the 16th chapter of the *Cikitsāsthāna*, *Kalpasthāna*, and *Siddhisthāna* in full; some portions are in verses while others are in prose. The styles are different in the portions composed by Caraka and Dṛḍhabala. According to his own statement, Dṛḍhabala is the son of Kapilabala and a resident of Punjab. The exact date and other details of his life and activities are yet to be known. He is believed to have lived before Vāgbhaṭa since he does not refer to him and so some scholars are of the opinion that he belonged to the third or the fourth century CE.

Sections in the Carakasamhita

There are 8 sections (*sthānas*) and 120 chapters in the *Carakasamhita*:

1. *Sūtrasthāna*
2. *Nidānasthāna*
3. *Vimānasthāna*
4. *Śārīrasthāna*

5. *Indriyasthāna*
6. *Cikitsasthāna*
7. *Kalpasthāna*
8. *Siddhisthāna*

The *sthānas* are divided again into chapters on the basis of the topic of discussion.

Of these, the first is the *Sūtrasthāna*; as the term denotes, it is like a thread (*sūtra*) that makes a garland of flowers, it binds together or gives an overall view of the content. This section presents the complete form of Āyurveda that is divided into cause, symptoms, and cure. There are 30 chapters in this *sthāna*; the first 28 chapters are divided into 7 groups:

1. *Bheṣaja*: gives details on medicines
2. *Svāsthya*: studies on health and moral conduct
3. *Nirdeśa*: instructs about treatments
4. *Upakalpana*: describes oleation, sudation, emission, and purgation.
5. *Rōga*: studies on ailments
6. *Yōjana*: describes formulation
7. *An̲n̲apān̲a*: explains compatible and incompatible diets, their transformation and assimilation.

The remaining two chapters are in the form of a summary. Topics such as the qualities of a physician are mentioned in these chapters.

Nidānasthāna, the second one, consists of eight chapters and describes important diseases in detail. The third is *Vimānasthāna*, which dilates on the *doṣa* (peccant humours). It discusses in eight chapters, various aspects of diseases, epidemics, causes of disorders, therapeutic strategies, nature of the four parts of the treatment, including the patient, the physician, the medicine and the helper or nurse, the individual nature of the human body, and so forth.

The fourth is *Śārīrasthāna*. The first chapter of this portion discusses the human being, and the *pañcabhūta*, the five elements that constitute his body, nature, mind, soul, and god in general. The following chapters discuss conception, development of limbs in the foetus, ways to beget a noble progeny, labour room, delivery, paediatrics, and so on. Though these studies are not elaborate, it provides adequate awareness for general medicine (*kāyacikitsa*).

Indriyasthāna, the fifth one, deals with symptoms of imminent death. This *sthāna* consists of 12 chapters. It says that a physician must be able to distinguish between diseases that can be cured and that cannot be; treatment can be effective only in the former cases. The physician identifies these symptoms through his sensual organs (*jñānendriya*), hence the title *Indriyasthāna*.

Cikitsasthāna, the sixth, has 30 chapters. The last 17 chapters are supplemented by Dṛḍhabala. Among these, the first two deal with rejuvenation (*rasāyana*) and aphrodisiac (*vājīkaraṇa*) therapies. The next six chapters follow the order as that of *Nidānasthāna*; then, from chapters 9 to 25, this order differs. This difference can also be seen in the chapters supplemented by Dṛḍhabala. However, from chapter 26 to 30 it is in the same order. The 30th chapter deals with the diet habits to be followed in different climates.

Kalpasthāna, the seventh one, deals with the method of preparation (*kalpana*) of medicines that induces vomiting (*vamana*) and purging (*virecana*) with their different forms. There are 12 chapters in this *sthāna* and so on.

The last one, *Siddhisthāna*, consists of 12 chapters; it deals with the likely errors that can occur in induced vomiting and purging, procedures to be adopted to rectify these errors and the effects of these treatments. It is clear from the above account that the text is meant for discussion of the various aspects of diseases and their treatment. True to the spirit of the Indian system of knowledge, the *Carakasamhita* upholds the importance of dharma, right conduct.

Caraka introduces the subject, stating that the knowledge on longevity has no limits; so, to promote this knowledge, one has to pursue the study constantly. He advises to accept noble thoughts from everywhere, even if it be from the enemy. Also, he directs that this science has to be imparted to the deserving, irrespective of the distinction of caste. All the four castes are entitled to this knowledge; the difference being in the aim. The Brahmin learns it to acquire the heavenly reward of holy and virtuous actions and for well-being, Kṣatriyas for the security of the subjects, Vaiśyas for livelihood, and Śūdra for service to others. Transmission of knowledge should be done after due verification; for knowledge, armoury, and water, passed on to the vicious, do harm to society. In learning and teaching this science, the preceptor, the disciple, and the science should be tested.

Qualities of a Disciple

The disciple should be noble, quiet, and good-looking; he should shun evil acts and should not be haughty. He should be intelligent, generous, interested, and inquisitive about the subject; balanced in mind and well-dressed. The student should be attentive and kind to all; he should treat happiness and misery alike. The disciple should have a sharp memory and should observe celibacy during the period of study.

Qualities of a Preceptor

The *ācārya*, the preceptor, must be well-versed in the texts, well-experienced, proficient, pure, and an expert in handling the subjects. Well-equipped and imaginative, he should know nature closely. An ideal preceptor would be kind to his disciples and interested in science and philosophy; he would be devoid of arrogance and anger; he would be kind in appearance and sturdy with the five senses; he should be dedicated, and teach with his penetrating insight that showers the bliss on his students. Like a favourable monsoon and fertile land yielding a rich produce, the rightly instructed student returns rich dividends.

Qualities of the Science

There are many prevalent medical sciences. What should be acquired is the one that is renowned, sought after by the learned, rich in meaning, adored by the dear ones, and universally intelligible. It should contain novel ideas and be composed by the ancient seers. Its merits should have stood the test of time; it should have commentaries and abstracts of aphorisms, and be informative and meaningful; it should have well-arranged chapters, and the contents should be defined with illustrations. Such a science dispels, like the sun, all the darkness around.

Initiation of the Disciple

The great preceptor imparts the noble science only to deserving disciples. The *ācārya*, after chants and libations in the presence of

Brahmins, physicians, and the holy fire as witnesses advises the student:

> Treat your patients sincerely; do not embarass them or quarrel with them even for sustenance. Never think of other women; clad yourself modestly. Never do or abet evil deeds; do only those things that suit the place and the milieu. Never accept food offered by women; visit a patient only after notification; walk with the head bowed. While visiting a patient's house do not let your heart, word or sense to digress. Keep the details of the patient confidential. Do not reveal to the patient or his relatives that death is approaching. If you deviate from these principles, may you be cursed and your learning becomes useless. If you behave improperly towards me or adopt means unbecoming the ethics of your profession, may your practice be barren and dull. Done properly this knowledge brings fame, friends and the goals of life to you. Serve the preceptor diligently as you serve fire, god, king and father.[6]

Prāṇābhisara

The knowledge of healthcare has two wings—theory and practice. One who knows the theory alone is puzzled before the patient like a coward in the battlefield. One who neglects the theory is like a one-winged bird. The one who is accomplished equally in theory and practice is always respected. He is known as the *prāṇābhisara*.

A discerning student will learn the name and identification of herbs and medicines from cowherds and jungle-dwellers. Practical study fulfils the knowledge of medicine. Physicians who have a sound knowledge of medicine and know how to administer it in accordance with the situation achieve success in their profession.

Dissection of the Body

The knowledge of anatomy is essential for a physician. This can be obtained by observing a dead body. The body dead due to poisoning or rotting diseases should not be used for this purpose. Remove excretion (*āntaramalas*) from the bowel and cover the corpse in grass and bark of trees to protect from insects, and immerse it in running water

[6] Varier, *History of Āyurveda*, 151.

The medicines must have the correct taste and smell. It should have no side effects or counter results if given mistakenly.

The helper is an essential part of the treatment procedure, especially in the cases of surgical operations and cases that require physical health for the physician and the patient. A helper must be reliable in confidential matters, friendly in behaviour, sincere in patient care, and physically strong. The helper should be hardworking, untiring, obedient, and sincere to the physician.

The patients are also expected to have some qualities for receiving treatment and completing it successfully. He should be endowed with the following qualities: He must have the physical capacity to receive treatment, he should have vitality, the disease must be curable, he must be endowed with the ability to procure articles for treatment, he should have self-control, and above all he must be ready to obey the physician.

Modalities of Treatment

The *Carakasamhita* has a list of guiding principles that consists of six plans of procedure. They are:

1. *Laṅghana* (lightening or slimming)
2. *Bṛāmhaṇa* (fattening or building)
3. *Rūkṣaṇa* (roughening)
4. *Snēhana* (lubricating)
5. *Svēdana* (fomenting)
6. *Stambhana* (arresting)

Langhana is prescribed for making the body lighter. *Bṛāmhaṇa*, building or fattening, is aimed at nourishing the body. In the case of fattening, the procedure starts with slimming slightly but those who are to be slimmed should not be fattened or nourished. *Rūkṣana*, roughening, is done for preparing the body to receive the treatment. Hardness, stability, sharpness, heat, coarseness, and lightness are qualities of the medication in this procedure. *Snēhana*, the lubricating procedure, is expected to moisten or soften the limbs and the body as a whole. *Svēdana*, fomenting, is meant for inducing sweat and for relieving stiffness. *Stambhana*, arresting, is done to arrest the flow of substances in the body channels (an example is given as constipation). This is expected to produce coldness, slowness, softness, roughness, stability, and so forth. In addition to these procedures, a set of five specific strategies are prescribed for eliminating the causes based on the loss of equilibrium of the *doṣas*.

Pañcakarma: The Five Evacuative Procedures

Vamana (emesis), *virecana* (purgation), *nasya* (nasal purging), *vasti* (enema), and *raktamokṣa* (blood-letting) are the *pañcakarma*, the five therapeutic strategies according to the Āyurvedic treatment procedure. Before starting the evacuative measures, including vomiting and so forth, the patient must have undergone lubricating and fomentation therapy. This is necessary for the body to receive the procedure. The patient should take bath, anoint the body, and should be properly dressed. The helper who is known to the patient should be ready always to help him. Sweetening may indicate the liquefaction of clogged *doṣas*.

Purgation is another evacuative procedure for which the drug must be chosen by the physician according to the patient's disorders, disposition, and location and time of other disorders. The signs of satisfactory purgation, post-purgation management, and the process of full recovery are similar to those of the emesis. Caraka most significantly notes that usually the protocol for *pañcakarma* befitted kings. But it should be made less costly and suitable, but no less effective for the poor too. If carried out properly, evacuative measures eliminate impurities, relieve illness, provide better strength, and prolong the life.

Nasya (nasal purging) is done if the disease is in the head. Two preparatory steps would be followed by an evacuative procedure in this. The medicine is taken through the nostrils to reach the inside of the head. This was generally performed once, twice, or thrice a day following a course of other procedures and lubricative therapy. The expected result includes the lightening of the head and chest, clearing of the senses, and the opEning up of the body channels. According to some Buddhist legend, this procedure was practised by the celebrated physician Jīvaka for a merchant's wife who was suffering from severe headache.[7]

[7] Zysk, *Asceticism and Healing in Ancient India*, 56.

Vasti or enema is regarded as a unique form of medical therapy used to evacuate unwanted elements quickly and easily in a procedure that is free from bad effects. It is held by experts that non-lubricant enema was superior to purgation. Two kinds of enema are the lubricant (*snēhavasti*) and non-lubricant (*kaṣāyavasti*). The non-lubricant is primary and the other one is secondary. Āyurvedic texts discuss in great details the indication techniques, equipments, special procedures, and so forth for the procedure. For obtaining specific effects, special drugs were added to the enema formulations.

According to Caraka, the non-lubricant enema, that is, *kaṣāyavasti*, is the best of all medical procedures. According to him, the order is non-lubricant enema, lubricant enema emesis (*vamana*), purgation (*virecana*), and nasal purging among the *pañcakarma*. Significantly, he does not consider blood-letting (*raktamokṣa*) though he was familiar with the strategy. This could be due to the reason that the procedures are based on a different result.

Contents of the *Carakasamhita*

Generally, Āyurvedic works have eight parts (*sthānas*) in 120 chapters, which contain the principal matters. The *Uttaratantra* or *Khilasthāna* is appended to deal with incidental matters. In the *Suśrutasamhita*, for example, surgery is dealt with in the main portion; and fever, inflammation resulting from wounds, and the cases of surgery of the eyes, ears, and nose, are dealt with in the *Uttaratantra*. Similarly, in the *Kāśyapasamhita*, the main portion deals with paediatrics and incidental diseases are considered in the *Khilasthāna*.

The number of chapters fixed as 120 is on the basis of the optimum lifespan of a human being.

The position of a physician was not hereditary. After completing the studies, on the advice of the preceptor, the student obtains royal permission. The preceptor examines his knowledge in theory and practice; he qualifies for the royal warrant only when recommended by another physician. The student should have deep learning in *tantra*, *tantrārtha* (the meaning of the *tantra*), *sthāna*, *sthānārtha* (the meaning of the *sthāna*), *adhyāya* (chapter), *adhyāyārtha* (the meaning of the chapter), *praśna* (problem), and *praśnārtha* (the meaning of the problem). The Gurukula system, staying and studying at the teacher's residence, was the mode of instruction followed in medical education. On completion of his studies, he is reborn as a physician. The story of Jīvaka narrated in the Buddhist texts illustrates the tests that a student had to pass through to become qualified.[8]

Dinacarya *(Daily Routine)*

The basis for the attainment of the goals of life, that is dharma (right duties), *artha* (right wealth), *kama* (right sensual pleasures), and *mokṣa* (eternal liberation from birth and death), is a sound mind in a sound body. Hence, Āyurveda gives prime importance to healthy and good living (*svasthavṛtta* and *sadvṛtta*); the non-observance of these principles causes diseases. The observance of ideal living is termed as *ācārarasāyana*. The traits of one who imbibes *rasāyana* (*rasāyanasevi*) are described in detail; and he attains the goal of life (*puruṣārtha*) who accomplishes all those characteristics.

Svasthavṛtta *(Health Routine)*

A strict routine is prescribed for a healthy life. One should wake up at the auspicious hour, that is, two-and-a-half hours prior to dawn, and start the daily routine (*dinacarya*); it includes ablutions and adornments which promote health, happiness, and elegance. While visiting patients, the *Suśruta* prescribes that physicians should wear clean white clothes and a turban; they must have footwear, a walking stick, and an umbrella. One must strive for prosperity, long life, and a happy afterlife; these can be earned through a regulated routine in daily life.

Physicians

Caraka speaks of three classes of physicians: pretentious (*chadmācāra*), accomplished in treatment (*siddhasādhaka*), and qualified (*guṇayukta*). However, they are mainly of two categories—*prāṇābhisaras* and *rogābhisaras*. The former are bestowers of life, with deep knowledge, experienced in theory and practice, experts, fully-equipped, knowing time and indications, noble and pure; they

[8] Zysk, *Asceticism and Healing in Ancient India*, 54–6.

drive diseases away and Caraka advises to bow and prostrate at the feet of such physicians.

But there are also some others who pretend to be experts and hang around patients' houses hoping for rewards. Whenever they hear of a sickness, they reach and plan to exploit the patient in all possible ways. Their technique is to condemn all other physicians and try to influence the friends of the patient. They conceal their ignorance very tactfully. The patient loses everything, but the ailment will not be healed. Then they begin to condemn the patient. When they realize that the patient is dying, they escape without being noticed and take a new name in another place. They shun the learned and impress fools with their own praises. They are *rōgābhisaras*, who spread diseases and the *ācāryas* warn against approaching them for treatment.

In this connection, it is significant to note that fake physicians make their appearance on the scene when a system of medical practice has developed into maturity and has become popular. They never like interactions with others; nor do they learn anything of their own. They have no preceptor, no disciples, or colleagues. Such physicians extend free entry of diseases into the body and take the life of the body; they are the messengers of death. Treatment for them is only a means of livelihood; like serpents they swallow life-giving air, and like hunters they trap patients in their nets. These are the characteristics of *rogābhisara* physicians. In this context, it is important to note that at the time of the redaction of the *Carakasamhita*, the system of Āyurveda was popular.

Social Life as Reflected in the Carakasamhita

Caraka gives us a glimpse of the state of society at the time of Jīvaka's teacher, Punarvasu Ātreya. Discussing the quest for wealth, Caraka suggests agriculture, cattle breeding, trade, and so on, as the means for acquiring the same. Musicians, instrumentalists, singers of invocatory verses, and narrators of legends and epics were popular among the people; other vocations are also described in different contexts. Interestingly, in addition to the four castes, he also mentions harlots, spies, numerologists, robbers, shopkeepers, and so on.

Instructions for baby care of those days are still relevant: children should not be frightened with the stories of a demon/giant (*rākṣasa*) and so forth; when selecting toys it should be harmless, safe, and devoid of sharp edges—(the *Kāśyapasamhita* mentions the names of toys); their dress should be washed daily, disinfected by fumigation with *guggulu* (*Commiphora mukul*), and the like. They should be kept clean, bathed, fed, and sent to sleep on time. Care should be taken in selecting nurses—they should be loving, healthy, and humble, of good disposition with unblemished character, and always clean.

Madyapāṉa *(Intoxication)*

Caraka lays down the rules for the consumption of meat and wine. He also describes marriage and *yajñas*. In the course of the Sautrāmaṇi sacrifice, devas drink wine (*sura*). The Sanskrit word for deva is *sura* as well. Caraka instructs *sura*—the splendour of Aśvinis, the energy of Sarasvati; called *rati* by man and ethereal beings (*gandharvas*, *yakṣas*, *rākṣasas*)—to be consumed in accordance with a certain method; and it prescribes the mode of consumption clearly. He prescribes meat to be taken with wine.

Wine, like food, causes diseases if used in excess; wine is compared to poison and cow's milk to energy. Wine vitiates *pitta*. Light (*laghu*), pungent (*tīkṣṇa*), hot (*uṣṇa*), sour (*amḷa*), reviving (*vyavāyi*), quick-acting (*āśukāri*), stringent (*rūkṣa*), prospering (*vikāśi*), and lucid (*viśada*) are the properties of wine. Caraka prescribes the use of wine as an anaesthetic during surgery and in labour intricacies.

In the context of eating meat, Caraka describes the merits of even cow meat. However, in other contexts he declares meat and wine as taboo. Scholars such as Deviprasad Chatopadhyaya point out that this contradiction is apparent for the ideas of different ages have crept into the work during its compilation.[9] Even according to the epics, Brahmins used to consume meat. But later, particularly after the advent of Buddhism and Jainism, the use of wine and meat became forbidden among Hindus. The approach of redactors might be influenced by the practices of these different stages and hence the contradiction.

[9] Deviprasad Chatopadhyaya, *Science and Society in Ancient India* (Amsterdam: B.R. Grüner, 1977).

Dhūmapāna *(Inhalation)*

In Caraka's time, *dhūmapāna* was a routine to be observed daily; in daily regimen (*dinacarya*) it was as prominent as ablution and so forth. Dhūmapāna is of three types, that is, practical (*prāyogika*), unctuous (*snaihika*), and purging (*vairecanika*). Eight different timings have also been instructed to do this. The length of the pipe may vary according to the type of *dhūmapāna*, the ingredients ground to a paste, smeared with medicine, and soaked in water, desiccated and cut in suitable lengths are to be used for inhalation. Different methods are instructed according to the diseases. Along with this, Caraka describes different types of fumigation (*dhūmāpanas*) for the disinfection of wounds and clothes. It specifies the points to be remembered in choosing friends; it stresses the good mental and physical health caused by living together with good friends.

Sex and Allied Matters

According to Caraka, the period for sexual activity is from 16 to 70 years of age. The marriageable age is 12 for girls and 21 for boys; the reproductive age is after 16 for females and 25 for males. Unapproachable women and amorous seasons are described in detail. Similar castes are preferred in union for good progeny. The bride should be of good physique, physiognomy, graceful, well-instructed, and obedient.

Women are to be respected and discourtesy towards them must be condemned. But, at the same time, Caraka warns not to trust them blindly, not to share confidential matters with them. While discussing the causes of the disease *raktagunma*, Caraka specially mentions the condition of women in that period. Women were dependent, uneducated, and always engaged in serving others. They get acquainted with blocking natural urges. Miscarriage, flatulence during menstruation, and so forth are the causes of *raktagunma* in women. Since their nature is tender like the aged and children, they should be administered only with gentle medicines.

Caraka restricts sexual activities according to seasons. It directs that one should mingle in a sexually indifferent manner with women in the summer, but permits complete sexual activity in winter and spring. Also, he says that one should not engage in conversation with strange women at a lonely place, or accept anything from a woman without her husband's permission.

Nursing Homes

Caraka describes the labour room (*sūtikāgāra*), the nursery (*kumāragṛha*), and the sweat room (*svedagṛha*). He also describes how to get into the hut especially made for *rasāyana* treatment (*kutīprāveśika*). He emphasizes that the labour house (*sūtikāgāra*) should be constructed over good floor that is free from bones, broken vessels, dust, sand, and so forth, and that all the necessary equipment should be stored properly. Caraka says that there will not be ailments in those houses that are built over an ideal place.

The site for such buildings should be safe from strong wind, birds, animals, reptiles, and rodents. It must be beautiful, bright, calm, and the one to which wind should come only from one direction. Suśruta describes the room for treatment of the wounded (*vraṇitāgāra*) with specific instructions. He directs that suitable places for the storage of water, closets, baths, kitchen, and so forth have to be allotted prior to the construction of the building. Beds, seats, linen, and so on should be so arranged that they can be used according to seasonal changes. The house for the sick must have servants, qualified and obedient, in addition to the necessary medicines and equipment for all types of treatment, including *svēdana* (sweating), *vamana* (vomiting), and so forth. A nursing home for treating the sick must have adequate precautionary means for handling emergencies.

Later epics and Buddhist literatures extol the construction of health centres as a noble act. Ashoka had provided facilities for free treatment of human beings, and animals in all parts of the country, including his own empire and outside it. The *Skandapurāṇa* and the *Nandipurāṇa* say that building such houses and providing medicine and so on through them are the most holy of all actions. Of all the gifts, the gift of life is the greatest. Fâ-hien (399–414 CE) describes the health centres of Pataliputra. Upanisa, the son of Buddhadāsa, built separate treatment centres for lepers, blind people, and pregnant women. According to Hsuan-tsang's report, Śīlāditya II built such centres in all towns and made provisions for free food and clothes. Such houses are often called holy homes, as they were open to all without the barriers of caste.[10]

[10] Zysk, *Asceticism and Healing in Ancient India*, 47.

Panorama of the Carakasamhita

According to Caraka, Āyurveda is a science whose scope is infinite; one must forever keep striving to acquire a thorough grasp of it. For the wise, the world is the preceptor; for fools the same is the enemy. Noble thoughts coming from anywhere ought to be listened to. What cures disease is the medicine; who relieves pain is the physician; the cure that does not lead to another ailment is the true treatment.

The science of treatment is as vast as the ocean, says Suśruta too. It cannot be explained even in a hundred thousand verses. No text can cover all the essentials. Hence, one should learn it directly from the preceptor. Learning one science does not make one accomplished; a physician is he who learns different sciences. Hence Āyurveda is associated with Sāṅkhya, Yōga, Nyāya, and other systems of philosophy. Its principles are also derived from worldly experiences. Mastery of many sciences broadens the intellectual horizon of a physician.

Rasāyana and *Vājīkaraṇa*

Rasāyana is rejuvenation, while *vājīkaraṇa* is the enhancement of virility, that is, sexual vigour. These are two integral parts of the programmes of treatment of Āyurveda. The *rasāyana* therapy is not an empty boast or a hollow advertisement but an effective procedure of treatment. Nor is it a programme aimed at arresting the ageing process. Instead, it is meant for preventing senile infirmities and miseries by appropriate measures adopted carefully to minimize the problems of ageing.

The term *rasāyana* has two parts: *rasa* and *ayana*. *Rasa* denotes the food sap from which the *dhātus* or the constituent elements of the body, such as blood, flesh, bone, marrow, semen, and so forth, are developed. This is the assimilable product of what is consumed as food and drinks. If *rasa*, the essence of food is insufficient, or if it is blocked, then it results in the replenishment of the *dhātus*. This is supposed to be the reason for ageing. *Ayana*, in this context, signifies the preparation of or smoothening of the routes of the food sap. Thus, *rasāyana* therapy is a method of assuring and augmenting the supply of *rasa* to the *dhātus* or the constituents of the body.[11]

[11] Valiathan, *An Introduction to Āyurveda*, 123–4.

Vāgbhaṭa observes that the best *rasāyana* is imbibing moral values, such as truthfulness, freedom from anger, inclination to spirituality, tranquillity, and benign acts. This amounts to saying that the intake of medical formulations without following an appropriate and lawful lifestyle cannot be expected to provide the desired result. In other words, Āyurveda insists that medicine and treatment provide the desired effect to those who observe noble ideals and lifestyle in their life. There are two modes of rejuvenation treatment: *kuṭīprāveśika* and *vātātapika*.

Kutīprāveśika insists that the treatment should be conducted in a house built especially for the purpose. The building facing north should have three concentric rooms with a small opening to provide access from one room to the other. The house must be well-protected from the hot sun, smoke, dust, beasts, and so forth. Women are prohibited from entering the house.

On an auspicious day, the treatment begins after having undergone the evacuative procedures. The subject should be free from all evil acts, words, and thoughts throughout the period of treatment. Then the *pañcakarma* programme begins. After the *pañcakarma*, the oral intake of the *rasāyana* begins according to the nature of the body of the patient in accordance with space and time. There are several formulations from which the physician chooses an appropriate one for the subject.

Vātātapika is the treatment for which special premises or protection from the weather and so forth are not prescribed. Moral values and right conduct are to be strictly followed and the usual preparatory procedures are to be conducted properly.

Vājīkaraṇa is meant for enhancing sexual potency. The term denotes the Āyurvedic measures to strengthen man to enjoy sexual intercourse with the virility of a horse. Prior to medication, the individual has to undergo purificatory measures and consume the prescribed diet of high nutrition value. The *vājīkaraṇa* therapy is also supposed to provide healthy offspring.

Caraka, Suśruta, and Vāgbhaṭa, the authors of the classical 'Great Triad',[12] are unanimous in emphasizing the importance of ethics in

[12] According to Musad, the 'Great Triad (*Bṛhtrayi*) of Āyurveda' is the *Carakasamhita*, the *Suśrutasamhita*, and the *Aṣṭāṅgahṛdaya* (K. Narayanan Musad, *Heritage of Healing* (CHS Souvenir, 2007), 112).

all human conduct, including sexual relations. Happiness in life, according to the *ācāryas*, lies in righteous conduct, that is, dharma.

Conceptual Considerations

The above-mentioned knowledge was conceptualized according to a system of enumeration, classification, and categorization. According to this system, all materials including the human body was constituted by *pañcabhūta*, five basic elements. They are:

1. *Pṛthvi*, earth
2. *Ap*, water
3. *Tejus*, fire
4. *Vāyu*, wind, and
5. *Ākāśa*, ether

The human body thus constituted is made up of seven *dhātus*, that is, basic building materials. They are:

1. *Rasa*, the sap
2. *Rakta*, the blood
3. *Māmsa*, the flesh
4. *Medas*, escessive fat
5. *Asthi*, the bone
6. *Majja*, the marrow, and
7. *Śukla*, the semen

The body thus created fall into three major *prakṛti*, natural groups. They are,

1. *Vāta*, the wind
2. Pitta, the bile, and
3. *Kapha*, phlegm

Treatment in the Āyurvedic system is for the *prakṛti* of the patient and not for the symptom or complaint of the disease.

Epistemology of Caraka

In Caraka's time, the sages speculated on various matters, such as the difference between timely and untimely death, the possibility of life after death, the source of life, the place for human effort in life, and so forth. Whatever is said on such matters in this work are considered to be the opinion of Punarvasu Ātreya. The philosophy in Caraka is autonomous and anterior to others. It does not accept the existence of God. Many contentions, such as *kālavāda* (explanation in thew concept of time), *svabhāvavāda* (explanation in the concept of character), and *sukhadukhavāda* (explanation in the context of happiness and sadness), discussed in the *Śāntiparva* of the *Mahābhārata* and the *Svetāśvataropaniṣad* are discussed in the *Carakasamhita* too. The philosophical underpinnings of the author are traceable mostly in the portions of the *Sūtrasthāna*, *Vimānasthāna*, and *Śārīrasthāna*. The author Caraka appears to be familiar with the concepts of *vyakta* (the clear), *avyakta* (the unclear), *prakṛti* (Nature), *puruṣa* (the personal self), *satva* (purity?), *raja* (dynamism?), and *tama* (darkness?). Similarly, he defines categories such as *dravya*, *guna*, *karma*, *samanyavisesha*, *samavaya*, and so forth of the Vaiśeṣika School of philosophy.[13]

Based on some concepts in the philosophy of yoga, some scholars argue that Caraka and Patañjali, the master of the yoga philosophy, are one and the same.[14] From a close look at the concepts in the philosophical treatise as well as in the work of Caraka, it can be understood that there are basic differences in the systems of Patañjali and Caraka. The most convincing evidence is in their treatment of the concept of yoga itself. Caraka describes yoga as the state of being free from the fetters of the mind (*antal̲ karaṇa*), such as happiness and misery, caused by *samsāra*, worldly life. In the *Śarīrasthāna*, he describes *puruṣa* as the union of *pañcabhūta*, the five basic elements and 24 principles. Patañjali describes two stages in the process of attainment of *mokṣa*. The first stage is the withdrawal of the mind from all external influences and concentrating on the self. This is the *samprajñāta* stage. The second stage represents the state of concentrating on the self in itself 'like a flame undisturbed by the wind'.[15] This is the *asamprajña* state of being. The emphasis here is on the detachment of the self from all other objects and the establishment of the self in its own effulgent state. Caraka does not identify two stages. Instead, his view of yoga is the restraining of the senses and the mind

[13] Jwala Prasad, *History of Indian Epistemology* (Delhi: Munshiram Manoharlal, 1987), 69–72.

[14] See Varier, *History of Āyurveda*, 91.

[15] Varier, *History of Āyurveda*, 97.

from external objects and concentrating the mind on the self. Yoga is the state in which all activities of the mind disappear on their own and never reappear. Setting of the mind and soul free from joy and sorrow is *mokṣa*. Caraka's yoga limits it with the *samprajñāta* stage and does not proceed to the stage of *asamprajña*. This is a basic difference between the two perceptions. There are other differences too regarding the objective of the yogic practice. Patañjali mentions even higher achievements such as *rithambhara, prajña,* and so forth. Thus, the objects of the two masters are different. They use different terminology and methods of explanation. In Patañjali, the powers are not eight as in the case of Caraka. He does not describe these powers as they obstruct the mainstream of yoga. In the fifth chapter of the *Sahimta* too, Ātreya is shown to distinguish between action and non-action and explains the importance of *satsaṅga*, mingling with noble people, and *brahmācārya*, celibacy, as means of attaining *mokṣa*, emancipation.

Contributions of Caraka

Caraka's most important contribution is the classical text of the *Carakasamhita* itself, which is the redacted and codified form of the *Agniveśatantra*, the source of the Samhita. It is in the *Carakasamhita* that we come across for the first time the basic concepts of Āyurveda, such as the theories of *tridoṣa, pañcabhūta,* and so forth, and similar philosophical concepts in their codified form with the necessary explanation. P.V. Sharma observes on the basis of a statement in the *Śārīrasthāna* (5.3) that it was Caraka who established the law of the uniformity of nature, which helped him apply the physical laws to the biological field.[16]

The traditional method of the *daivavyapāśraya* (divine) mode of treatment was replaced by the *yuktivyapāśraya* (empirico-rational) therapy with the codification of the *Carakasamhita*. This change was brought in by incorporating the theory and methods of heterodox sects of Jaina and the Buddhist *saṅgha*s too into the healing and healthcare system while retaining the invaluable knowledge and practices of Vedic medicine. Thus, it may be observed that the *Carakasamhita* was keen in retaining the ideas of tradition and

16 Sharma, *Caraka Samhita*, xxvii.

modernity. Caraka's emphasis was on the process of investigation, which is essential for arriving at scientific truth, and hence he repeatedly uses the word *parīkṣa* (test) instead of *pramāṇa* (source).

One of the instituted methods prescribed for the advancement of knowledge and research was discussion among experts. Symposia were organized in different places for achieving this end.[17] Caraka alludes to one such occasion in verse 12 of the *Sūtrasthāna* where he presents a list of great *ācāryas* who 'gathered in one of the auspicious sides of Himalaya' and participated in the discussions. It was these exchanges of ideas that were instrumental in developing broader scientific perspectives, which led to the study of various problems of medicine and its use from different angles to arrive at the truth.

Caraka was responsible following the psychosomatic approach in understanding the human body and its nature. The treatise holds the synthetic view instead of analysing it into numerous parts and reducing it to an aggregate of innumerable cells. According to the *ācārya*, body and mind interact mutually and, therefore, disorders in the human body are to be viewed accordingly. This is known among the experts as the *dehanmānasa*, meaning psychosomatic principle.

Following closely the philosophic world view of the Vaiśeṣika School, Caraka emphasized the importance of the psychic and somatic constitution of the human body. This is what is known as the *prakṛti*, which became the centrality of treatment.[18] According to this view, every individual is endowed with his own particular nature and normal variations. This is the base for his *prakṛti*, constitution, which distinguishes him from other fellow beings.

The traditional method of the threefold *hetu-liṅga-auṣdha* (cause-gender-ailment) principle was further analysed and elaborated into the fivefold principle of *nidāna-pūrvarūpa-rūpa-upaśaya-samprāpti* (cause-earlier form-form [present]-remedy-the path of vicious effect). This became the five means of *parīkṣa*, investigation and diagnosis of diseases. The method provided a strong scientific base for the whole procedure of treatment. Further, it was instrumental for the expansion of the whole discipline of Āyurveda.

The *Carakasamhita* provided a scientific method of diagnosis of diseases by examining various aspects such as *doṣa*, *dūṣya* (malignancy),

[17] *Carakasamhita*, *Sūtrasthāna*, 1: 6, 7.

[18] For details, see the section on 'Epistemology of Caraka' on p. 45.

agni (fire), *sattva* (basic object), *sātmya* (similarity), *prakṛti* (nature), *balavayas* (age), and so on. Caraka prescribed a systematic procedure of the 10 entities to be examined before proceeding to the treatment. Aetiology, symptoms, suitability, and pathogenesis are to be examined before proceeding to action.

Nature was attributed with utmost importance for providing proper assistance to it. Medicine and other therapeutic measures are all for curing the disorder of the patient. Promotion of life by preventing ailments was prescribed as the final goal of treatment. Thus, Caraka emphasized the importance of dharma by giving several formulas. This is what is known as the *swasthavṛtta* and *dinacarya*.

A thorough knowledge of plants with respect to name, form, properties, action, and therapeutic uses is essential for a physician since it was the most important material for treatment. Information about various aspects had been accumulating from the Vedic period onwards. Systematic codification of this important knowledge is perhaps one of the most important contribution of *Carakasamhita*.[19] In addition to this, the text codifies the existing knowledge of the basic concepts of pharmacology, including the five aspects—*rasa*, *guṇa* (quality), *vīrya* (strength), *vipāka* (change/transformation), and *prabhāva* (effect).

What is given above is a brief account of the most valuable contributions of Caraka, who is considered to be one of the fountainheads of the knowledge of Āyurveda. However, we confess that it is only a primary note that may be further expanded by carefully enumerating the rich and varied scientific aspects of the entire treatise of Caraka.

[19] For a detailed account of this aspect, see *Sūtrasthāna*.

4

Suśrutasamhita

Suśruta is widely known as the ancient Indian authority of surgery and as the author of the *Suśrutasamhita*, the authentic text of surgery. The celebrated author studied under Divodāsa, the king of Kāśi, and he was a descendent of Dhanvantari who must be different from the celebrated physician of the royal court of Chandragupta Vikramāditya. The story relates how he was selected by his fellow students to put questions to the *ācārya* Divodāsa and also to explain the difficult ideas in the *ācārya*'s answers to them. As usual, Suśruta's date is a subject of unending debate. The period attributed to him ranges between 1000 BCE to 700 BCE. Some scholars are of the opinion that the great surgeon was later than Jīvaka, the celebrated physician who, according to tradition, treated the Buddha, the Enlightened One.

Suśruta's date is, as usual, a subject of controversy. He is assigned by a section of scholars to a period as early as 1000 BCE and this is on the basis of a reference to his name in Panini's *Aṣṭādhyāyi*. The great grammarian is generally dated to circa seventh century BCE on the basis of speculations. At the same time, it may be noted that an aphorism in the treatise (4, 1: 49) refers to *yavanani* (the Greeks), whose presence in the north-west cannot be earlier to 519, with reference to the Bahistun inscription of Darius, which includes Gandhara in his empire. A mature system of writing and a developed language implied by the treatise tentatively indicate around fifth century BCE as the earliest date for the great grammarian. Therefore, Suśruta can be taken to have lived in the sixth century BCE. At the same time, his treatise *Suśrutasamhita*, the classical text of surgery, in its present form appears to belong to a much later date. This is a logical inference based on the subject matter of the text. In the initial portion, the preceptor Divodāsa mentions *rasāyana* and *vājīkaraṇa* as two therapeutic strategies for a long life and sexual virility. These were aspired to especially by a pleasure-seeking leisurely section of society which appeared in the peak period of urbanization around the beginning of the Common Era.

Suśrutasamhita

The *Suśrutasamhita* discusses all the important topics in 120 chapters divided into five *sthānas*: *sūtra*, *nidāna*, *śārīra*, *cikitsa*, and *kalpa*. The *Uttaratantra* is like an appendix; some scholars are of the opinion that the word suggests something added to the main body. The focus in the *Suśrutasamhita* is on surgery and, therefore, the *cikitsāsthāna* begins with a discussion on surgery. Keeping in mind the overall aim and objectives of Āyurveda, it goes on to deal with the prevention of inherent diseases and methods for maintenance of health. The text lays down specific procedures for studying the science of surgery and describes various aspects of the topic of surgical treatment. Here, the author describes in great detail different types of instruments used for surgery—for cutting and opening parts of the body. The mode of cutting is categorized as *chedya* (excision), *bhēdya* (incision), *lekhya* (scraping), *vēdhya* (puncturing), *ēśya* (probing), *āharya* (extracting), *visrāvya* (drainage or evacuation), and *seevya* (suturing).

Surgical instruments known as *yantras* and *śastras* are mentioned in detail. One hundred and one implements are described here. The names of these instruments, such as *simhamukha*, *vyāghramukha*, *kākamukha*, and so forth, suggest a high degree of expertise in metallurgy, and this is also a pointer to the period of the text. Apart from actual sugery, some other stategies also find mention in the text. These include *kṣāra* or alkalis, burning, and *raktamokṣa* or blood-letting.

Sūtrasthāna

The first chapter deals with treatment in a nuclear form; this is amplified in later chapters. As in the *Carakasamhita*, the disciple has to undergo severe tests before initiation. Physical contact, even coming nearer, was taboo. Suśruta prescribes in detail the nature of labour rooms and the furniture and so forth. The text recommends feeding of 1,000 Brahmins in that particular period. The privileges and preferences allowed to Brahmins indicate in unequivocal terms the supremacy enjoyed by them during the period of the compilation of the text. This may be of some help for the discussion of the date of the author of the text. However, one does not know whether these portions are later interpolations.

Suśrutasamhita gives equal importance to theory as well as practice. He says that medicine, an elixir for life, can be like poison in the hands of the inept. Like Caraka, Suśruta too emphasizes the need for mastery over many disciplines. He states that the science should be learnt from the preceptor; learning from books alone is like stealing.

Surgery is set in three phases, namely *pūrvakarma* (pre-operative treatment), *pradhānakarma* (treatment), and *paścātkarma* (post-operative treatment). *Pūrvakarma* means preparation, of both patient and the instruments, before the operation; *pradhānakarma* means the surgery proper; and *pascātkarma* means the treatment after the operation.

It is understood from the *Suśrutasamhita* that anaesthetics were not in use, but intoxicants were given to reduce the pain. The qualities of a good surgeon and the points he must have to bear in mind are described in detail. Patients were given a light diet, except in abdominal surgery. It tells us that the surgical instruments should move along the fibre avoiding bones, joints, blood vessels, nerves, and plexuses as far as possible.

Tools and instruments

A large variety of instruments were used for surgical operations. According to some recent scholars, Suśruta's outstanding achievement is the 'design, development and appropriate use of a large variety of surgical armamentarium'.[1] The surgical tools designed by Suśruta included 100 blunt instruments and 20 sharp ones. The blunt instruments were used for removing foreign objects from the body, such as arrow heads and similar sharp things. These tools, differently

[1] Valiathan, *An Introduction to Ayurveda*, 101.

identified as *simhamukha* (lion-mouthed), *vyāghramukha* (tiger-mouthed), *sṛgālamukha* (jackal-mouthed), and so forth, were fabricated by skilled blacksmiths. Another variety of instruments was meant for extracting deep-seated foreign bodies and they were designed resembling the beaks of birds, such as eagle, heron, crow, and so forth. There were also instruments in this category, including a pitcher forceps, and tubular and rod-like tools. The sharp instruments included different varieties of knives, scissors, needles, hooks, and so forth. He ordained that the tools must be made by skilled blacksmiths, and also that a surgeon must be in constant touch with the instruments since his success depended on the skilled use of the apt instrument in the appropriate manner. The text mentions 101 surgical instruments; the hand is the most important one among them. The numbers may vary, as the operations are many. They are grouped under six types: (*a*) *svastik*-24, (*b*) *tala*-2, (*c*) *salaka*-28, (*d*) *sandamśa*-2, (*e*) *nāḍi*-20, and (*f*) *upayantra*-25. The artistic style of these tools and implements clearly indicate a high rate of metallurgical skill on the part of the metal workers (Figure 4.1).

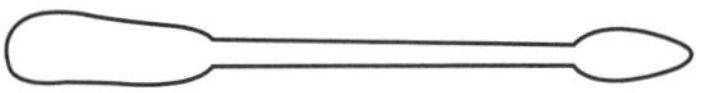

i. Trocar (*vrīhīmukha*)

ii. Awl (*ārā*)

iii. Double-edged knife (*vetasapatraka*)

iv. Sharp hook (*baḍiśa*)

v. Dental scaler (*dantaśaṅku*)

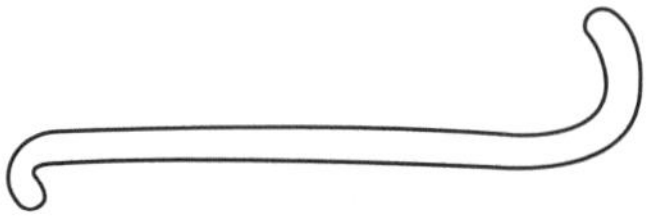

vi. Probes (*esaṇi*)

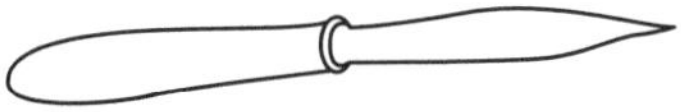

vii. For drainage of abscess (*kuśapatra*)

viii. For drainage of abscess (*āṭīmukha*)

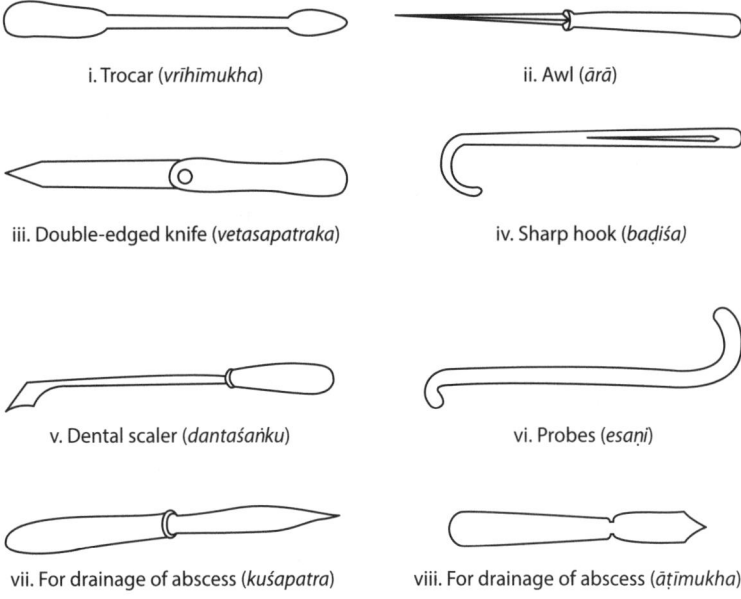

Figure 4.1 Surgical Tools
Source: Ayurveda College, Kottakkal.

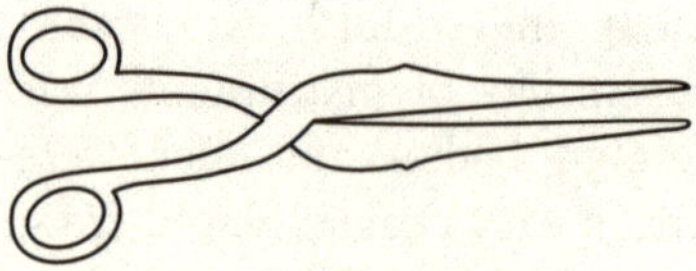

ix. Mouth like *śarāri* bird
(*śarārimukha*)

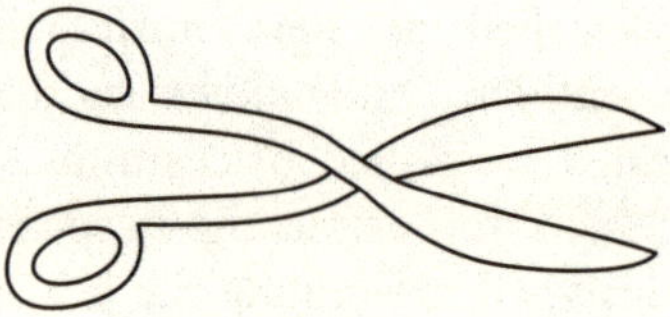

x. Semi-lunar–shaped scissors
(*antarmukha*)

xi. Three-bladed instrument
(*trikūrcaka*)

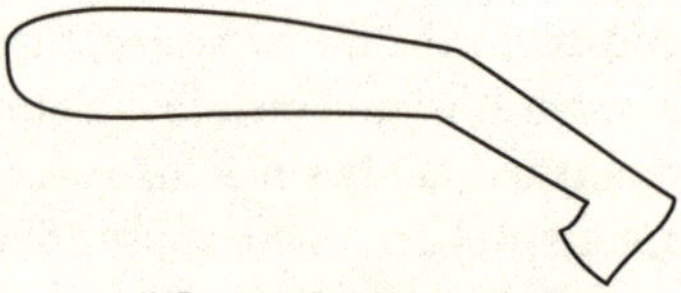

xii. Puncturing instrument
(*kuṭhārika*)

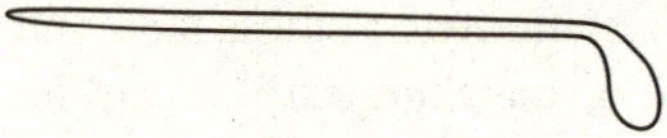

xiii. Jamul seed–like probe
(*jāmbavavadana* or *jāmbavauṣṭha*)

xiv. Bud-shaped (*mukuḷāgra*)

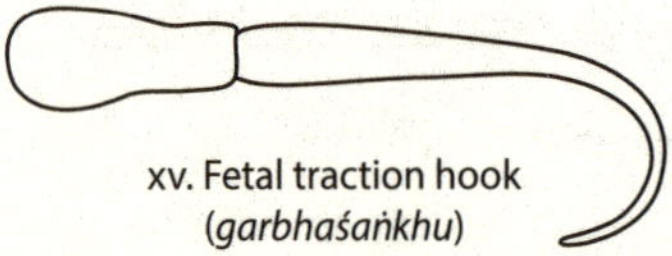

xv. Fetal traction hook
(*garbhaśaṅkhu*)

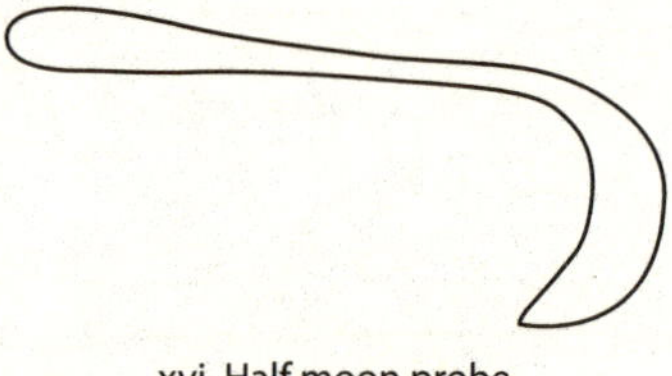

xvi. Half moon probe
(*ardhacandramukha*)

xvii. Earthworm-like probe
(*gaṇḍūpadamukha*)

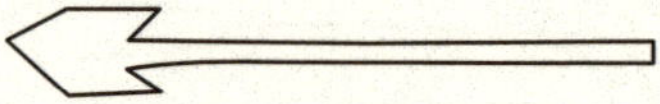

xviii. Arrow-wing–like
(*sarapuṅkhamukha*)

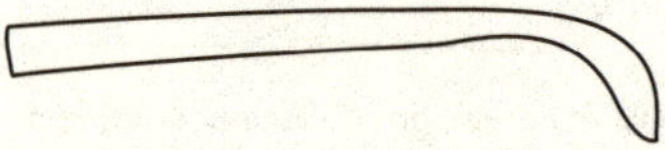

xix. Snake-hood-like (*sarpaphaṇamukha*)

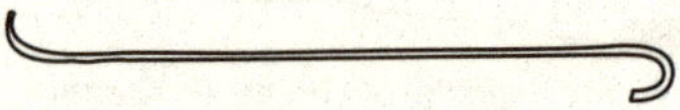

xx. Fish-hook–like (*baḍiśamukha*)

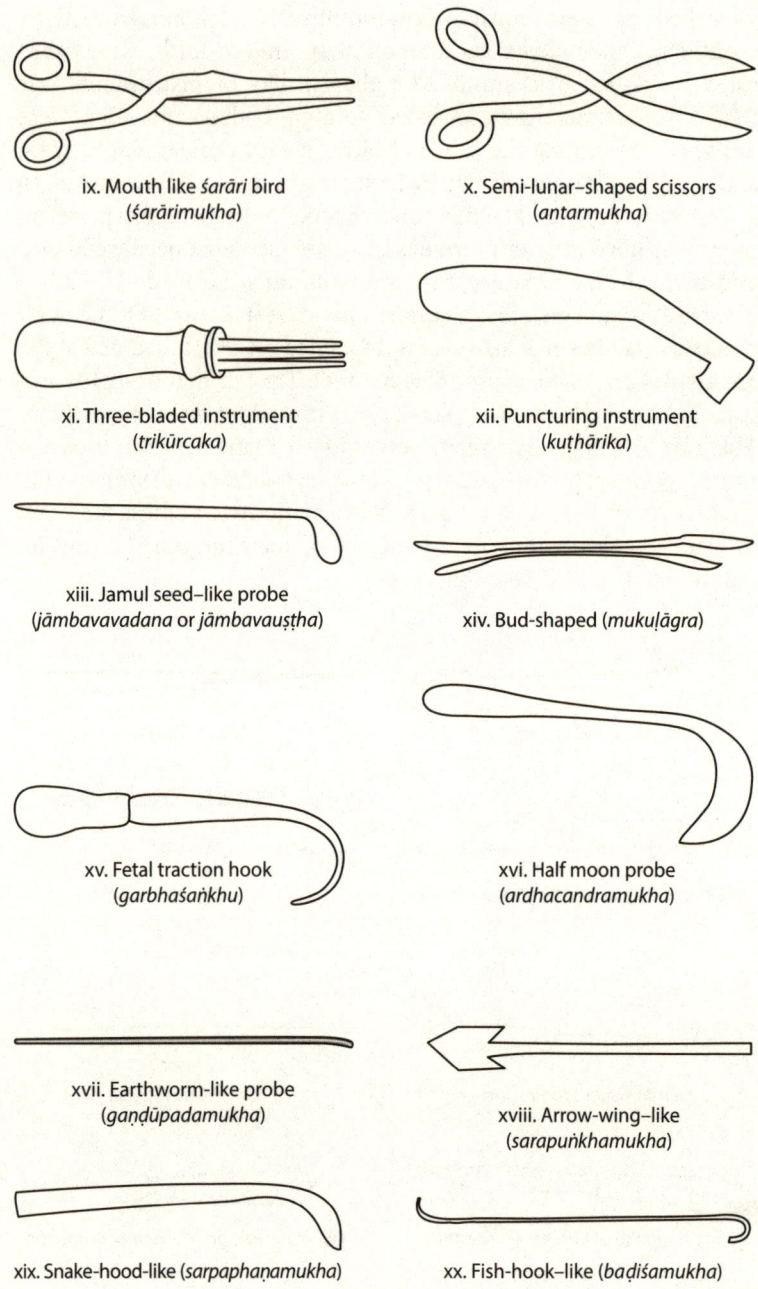

Figure 4.1 (*Cont'd*)

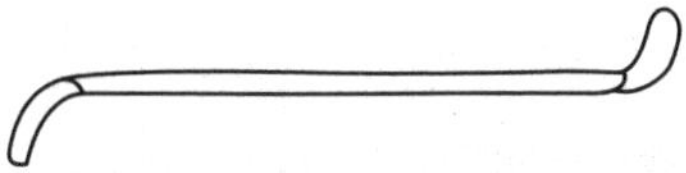

xxi. Lentil pulse–like (*masūnradaḷamukha*)

xxii. Swab-holding probe (*pramārjana*)

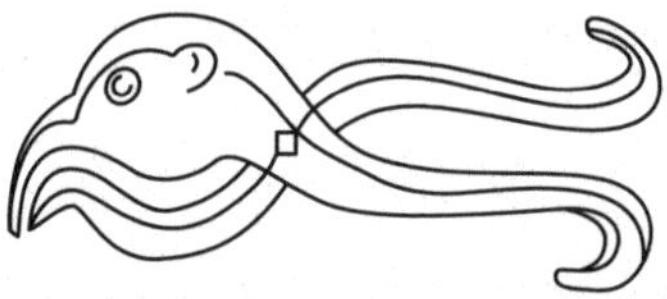

xxiii. Owl forceps (*ulūkamukha*)

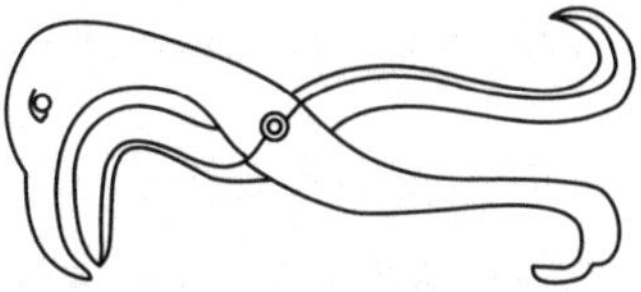

xxiv. Kite forceps (*cillīmukha*)

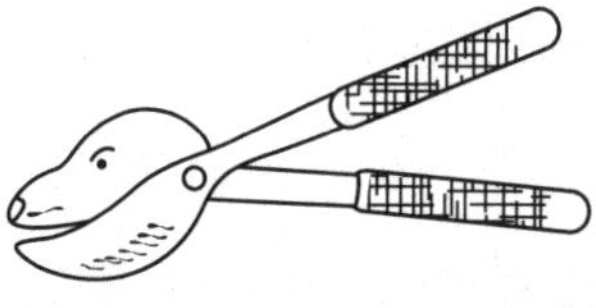

xxv. Vulture forceps (*śyenamukha*)

xxvi. Falcon forceps (*gṛdhramukha*)

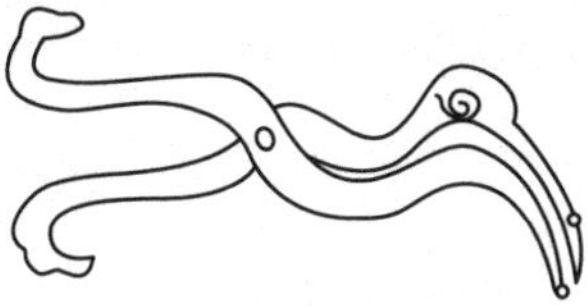

xxvii. Curlew forceps (*krauñcamukha*)

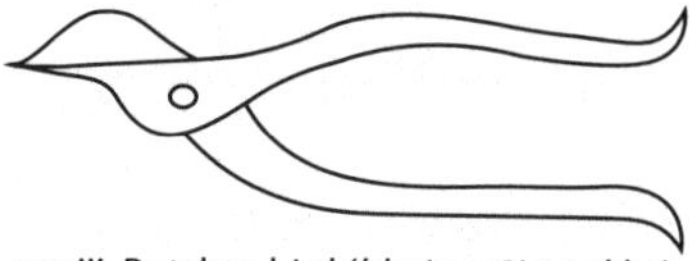

xxviii. Butcher-bird (*bhṛṅgarājamukha*)

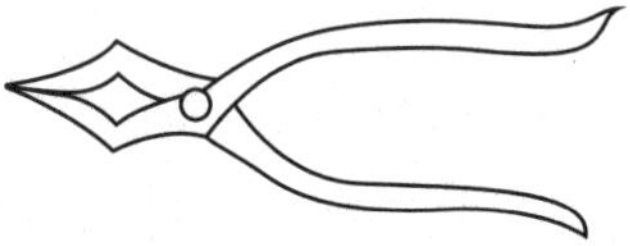

xxix. With arms

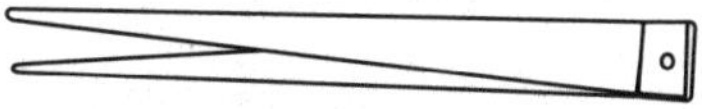

xxx. Without arms

xxxi. Single blade (*ekatala*)

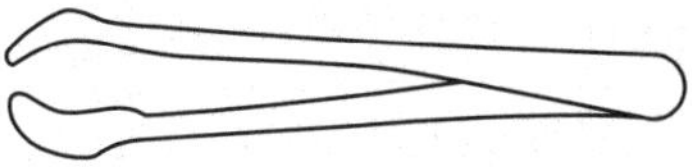

xxxii. Double blade (*dvitala*)

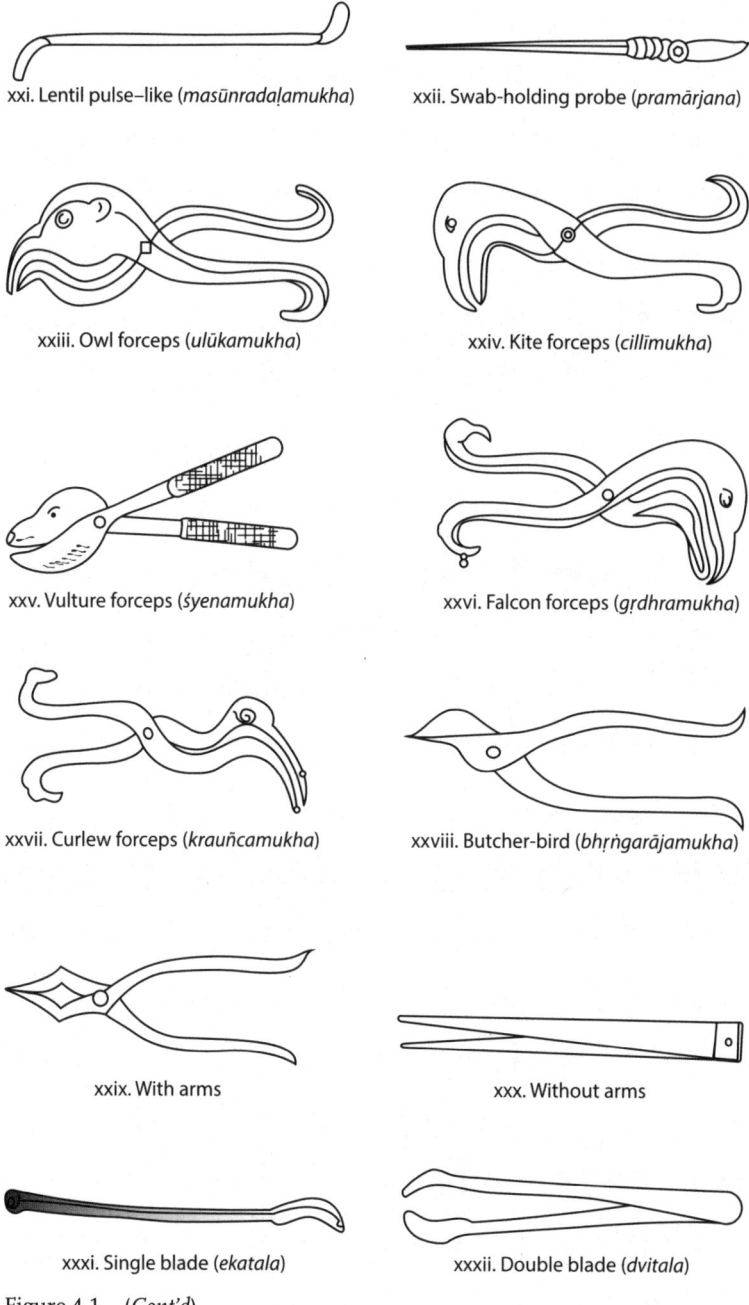

Figure 4.1 (*Cont'd*)

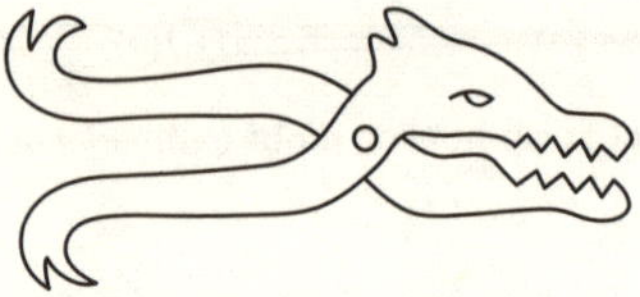

xxxiii. Jackal face (*sṛgālamukha*)

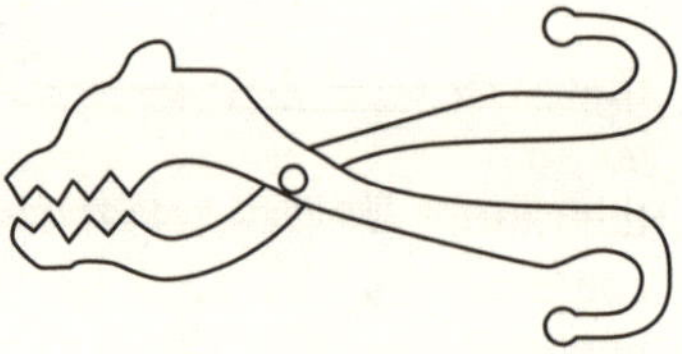

xxxiv. Cat face (*mārjāramukha*)

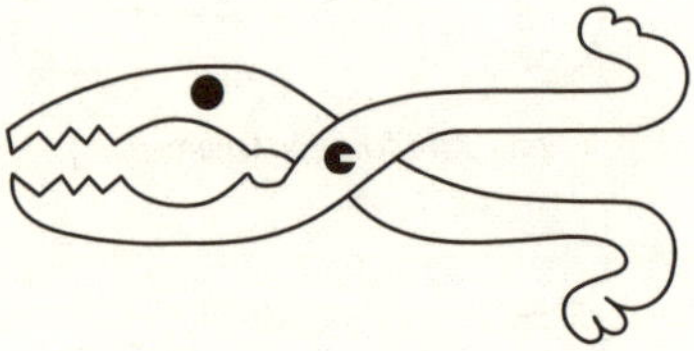

xxxv. Panther face (*dvīpīmukha*)

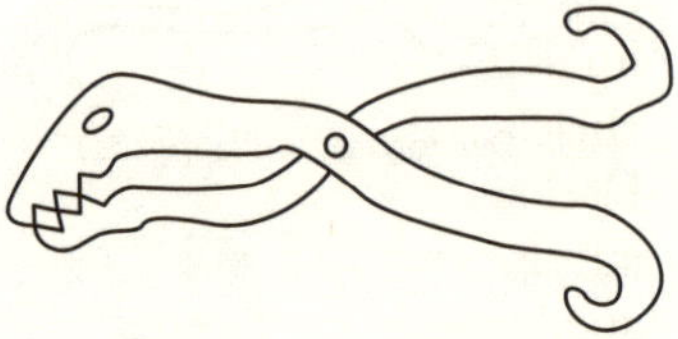

xxxvi. Deer face (*ervārukamukha*)

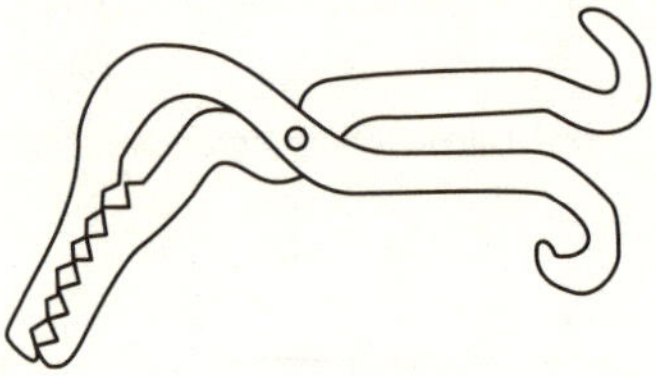

xxxvii. Crocodile face (*makaramukha*)

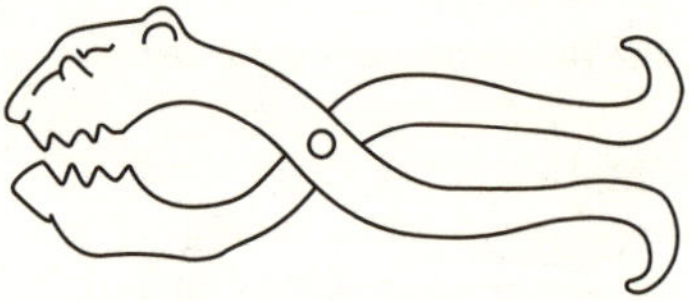

xxxviii. Lion face (*simhamukha*)

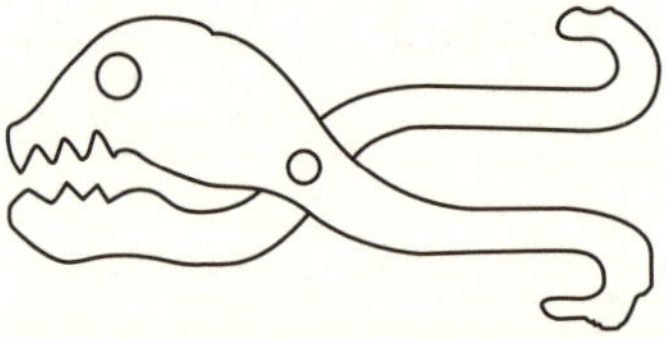

xxxix. Tiger face (*vyaghramukha*)

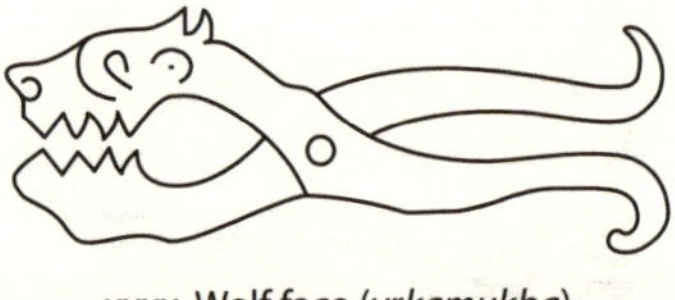

xxxx. Wolf face (*vṛkamukha*)

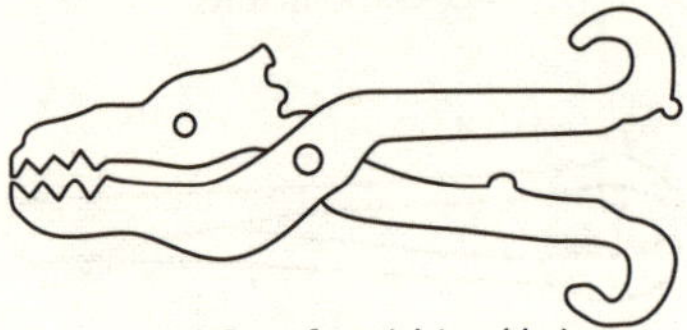

xxxxi. Bear face (*ṛkśmukha*)

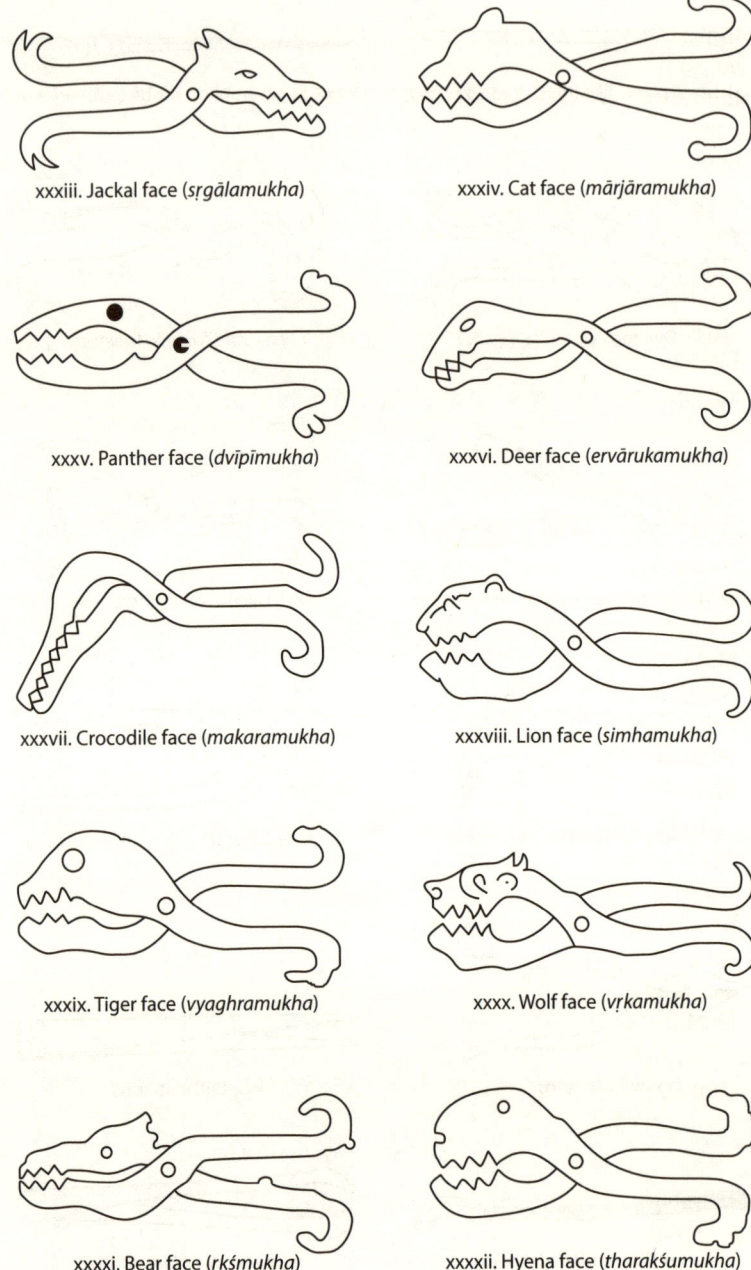

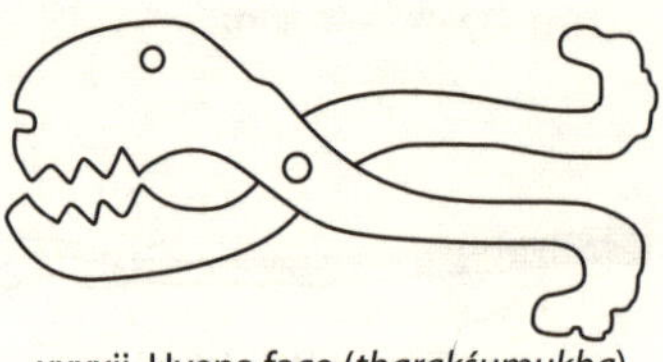

xxxxii. Hyena face (*tharakśumukha*)

Figure 4.1 (*Cont'd*)

These tools and implements are historically important in that they imply a high rate of metallurgical skills in their making. The cultural importance of these materials becomes clear only against their technological background. In spite of the scarcity of sources, one could attempt some kind of speculation thanks to the limited data obtained from well-defined layers of early iron-age sites in India. Scholars have identified the middle of the first millennium BCE as an early phase of the NBP archaeology, which witnessed the proliferation of tools for specialized jobs, such as sickles and spades for agricultural purposes; the smith's anvil and tong; crucibles, drills, adzes, chisels, and knives for carpenters; and moth pieces of bellows for blacksmiths. This is taken as clear indication of an agricultural surplus required for the development of specialized metal craft. This sudden efflorescence in iron-working at some sites is indicative of a quickening phase of urbanization.[2]

In north-western India, iron appears in the Gandhara Grave culture, which is dated from the ninth to the sixth century BCE. The recorded objects included spearheads, nails, spoons, flat rectangular axes, parts of horse furniture, such as the cheek bar of the horse's harness, and so forth. In central India, including the Tapti Valley and Malwa, iron started appearing from the Period II sites, such as Nagdha, Prakash, Bahal, Eran, and so forth. This culture is dated around 1000 BCE. A later layer is characterized by the association of Painted Grey Ware (PGW), which began with the earliest use of iron in the Ganga valley. The types of objects of iron from this phase include, apart from slag, some arrowheads, spearheads, knife, nails, spade, crowbar, dagger, hoe, fishhook, tong, and adze. This is dated with the supporting date from around 1000 to 600 BCE. The political history of this phase began with a number of territorial units, each of them politically centralized, extensive craft specialization, and a considerable amount of trade and commerce.[3] Archaeologists who are familiar with the stratified materials from the excavated trenches are of the opinion that the available data seems to indicate that the use of iron became an all-encompassing technology with the beginning of

[2] T.N. Roy, *A Study of Northern Black Polished Ware* (Delhi: Ramanand Vidyabhavan, 1986), 187–8.

[3] Dilip K. Chakrabarti, 'Beginning of Iron and Social Change in India', in *Iron and Social Change in Early India*, ed. Bhairabi Prasad Sahu (Delhi: Oxford University Press, 2011), 114–20.

this historical epoch. Significantly enough, N.R. Banerjea lists as many as 28 objects against the 14 of an earlier listing.[4]

Fumigation with *guggulu* (*Commiphora mukul*), *agaru* (*Aquilaria agallocha*), *sarjarasa* (*Shorea robusta*), mustard, salt, and neem (the leaf of *Azadirachta indica*), mixed with ghee, was advised for the disinfection of wounds. The administration of ghee, orally or by massaging, was advised to regain the consciousness of the patient; after that, safety measures against reinfection and evil spirits were adopted. The patient was then advised on diet and regimen. The dressing was untied on the third day and after that medicines, diet, and so on, were decided based on the strength and age of the patient. The *Suśrutasamhita* describes wounds, clean and unclean, and their symptoms of healing in detail. The possibilities of being cured, things to be avoided, precautions in dangerous situation, and so forth are also described.

The climate plays an important role in the treatment as well as in the collection of herbs, which, out of season, might lack quality and even be harmful. Polluted medicines and diet may cause illness and lead even to death; therefore, the seasons, seasonal duties, and precautions are all explained in the Samhita.

There are 20 instruments for the eight types of surgical operations. The ways to store them carefully, and maintain their sharpness, methods of their practice, and so on are also explained in detail. The disciple, after becoming adept in theory and practice, is sent off for setting up his own practice. Like Caraka, Suśruta also prescribes a code of conduct to the physicians.

Apart from the above instruments, the text explains other important means of cure, such as alkalis, cauterization, and the use of leeches in extracting impure blood. It advises the treatment of some minor cases with alkalis. These alkalis, prepared out of various medicines, normalize the imbalance of the three humours (*tridoṣa*). Alkalis for internal use are known as *paniya* and for external use as *pratisaraṇīya*.

It states that cauterization (*agnikarma*) is more powerful than alkalis (*kṣārakarma*); the cure in this case will be permanent. Cauterizations are resorted to when medicine, surgery, and alkalis fail. Many types of materials used for cauterizations, such as long pepper,

[4] N.R. Banerjea, *The Iron Age in India* (Delhi: Munshiram Manoharlal, 1965). See also Dilip K. Chakrabarti, 'Beginning of Iron in India: Problem Reconsidered', in *Perspectives in Palaeo-anthropology*, ed. A. K Ghosh (Calcutta, 1973), 345–56.

excreta of goat, teeth of cows, metals, honey, ghee, jaggery, and the like have been discussed in detail. The four types of cauterizations and their signs—adequate, inadequate, and over application—are also explained.

Leeches are used for blood-letting for those who are wary of pain and are weak. There are two kinds of leeches—toxic and non-toxic. Details regarding their collection, cleaning, application, relieving, and maintenance for further use are available in the text. As an effective treatment, it recommends blood-letting for many cases.

Long earlobes are said to be a sign of beauty. The stretching of earlobes for wearing ornaments and the resultant ailments and their treatment are described in it; the grafting of flesh from nearby areas in such cases and the grafting of a damaged nose in a similar way are also explained. India was the pioneer in this art and it spread to other countries from here. These portions in the text are extremely interesting since they shed much welcome light on various historical aspects including the nature of punishments.

Suśruta describes the causes, development, and cure of ailments in a graceful style. The humours (*dōṣas*) accumulate in their respective areas. When vitiated, they spread to other areas, interact with other *doṣas*, and intermix with blood; this action develops in 15 different ways. Diseases appear with clear symptoms after this. It is said that there are six phases for the cause of diseases, namely accumulation, vitiation, diffusion, inter-mixture, initial revelation, and outburst; it would not develop if tackled at the stage of accumulation. Suśruta states that treatment should be in the order of the accumulation of humours involved; first the disorders have to be brought under control.

Diseases are of seven types:

1. inherited (*ādibalapravṛtta*), for example, leprosy and piles.
2. congenital (*janmabalapravṛtta*), for example, deafness, blindness, and deformity.
3. imbalance in humours due to improper habits (*doṣabalapravṛtta*), for example, fever and dysentery.
4. seasonal (*kālabalapravṛtta*), for example, diseases due to seasonal changes.
5. superhuman (*daivabalapravṛtta*), for example, diseases due to witchcraft and cursors.
6. natural (*svabhāvabalapravṛtta*), for example, due to hunger, thirst, old age, and so forth.

7. incidental (*saṅghata balapravṛtta*), for example, diseases due to external causes, such as attacks by wild animals, weapons, and so forth. However, it says that the basic reason for all these seven groups is *tridoṣa*.

What displeases the body and the mind is called a disease and the 'treatment' is to assuage them. Lust, anger, greed, and so forth irritate like an arrow that is lodged in the flesh; 15 ways are prescribed to get rid of them, namely (*i*) nature (*svabhāva*), (*ii*) suppuration (*pacana*), (*iii*) excision (*bhedana*), (*iv*) cleaving (*dāraṇa*), (*v*) pressing (*pīḍana*), (*vi*) cleansing (*pramārjana*), (*vii*) sucking (*nirddhmāpana*), (*viii*) emesis (*vamana*), (*ix*) purgation (*virecana*), (*x*) flushing (*prakṣāḷana*), (*xi*) snuffing (*pratimarśa*), (*xii*) enema (*pravahaṇa*), (*xiii*) probing (*cūṣaṇa*), (*xiv*) magneto therapy (*ayaskānta*), and (*xv*) exhilaration (*harṣa*). Suśruta states that treating fatal diseases may bring a bad name to the physician; some symptoms of impending death (*riṣṭas*) are also explained in detail. The descriptions on treatment procedures are almost the same as in Caraka. The appropriate method of treatment according to *Suśruta* is to deal with the most prominent and provoked disorder without exciting the others.

Suśruta analyses in detail the world as a composite of *pañcabhūta*, the five basic elements. All materials are composites of *pañcabhūta* and so are medicines; they differ only in their proportion. The *bhūta*s, like earth and water, have a dense nature and tend to gravitate downwards and hence become purgatives; so, purgative drugs are the ones chosen from those with the predominance of earth and water. Drugs having a predominance of fire, ether, and air are used to induce vomiting, as those tend to move upwards. Suśruta says that knowledge about herbs is to be obtained from cowherds, jungle-dwellers, and hermits and from those who live on jungle produce.

The author describes the substances that are useful in healing wounds and categorizes them as: (*i*) anti-inflammatory (*śophaharaṇa*), (*ii*) cleaving drugs (*dāraṇadravya*), (*iii*) pressing drugs (*pīḍana-dravya*), (*iv*) purgative ghee (*saṃśodhanaghṛta*), (*v*) purgative oil (*samśodhanataila*), and (*vi*) incensing drugs (*dhūpanadravya*). The chapter 'Dravyasaṅgrahaṇīya' gives a classification of all raw materials.

Generally, there are two approaches of treatment in Āyurveda: (*i*) purification, that is, the elimination of harmful substances from the body (*samśodhana*), and (*ii*) pacification, that is, mollifying harmful substance internally (*samśamana*). It is said that the *śodhana cikitsa* is more preferable as it deters the regeneration of harmful substance, whereas after the *śamana cikitsa*, the doubts of regeneration of the *doṣa* persist.

Suśruta's method of arriving at definite conclusions in practical and theoretical issues is interesting. He discusses various theories and thoughts prevalent among the *ācāryas* of his time regarding the problem under consideration and finally gives his own conclusions. Unlike Caraka, he does not mention an *ācārya* by name.

The descriptions of food and drink in the *Suśrutasamhita* are based on the classification of solids and liquids. The quality of water, its source and purification, method of collection, cooling and storage, and so forth are explained in detail; a description of the rivers of India is also given in this portion. It also describes the properties of river water. Fast-flowing river water will be light; slow-flowing river water will be impure and stagnant; water with moss will be heavy; water in the river of desert will have a salty taste. *Aṣṭāṅgahṛdaya* also holds the view that water flowing through rocky areas will be light. The description then passes on to other liquids such as milk, curd, and urine groups.

Suśrutasamhita categorizes and defines the items that are good for consumption in the chapter on dietary regimen (*an̲n̲apān̲avidhi*). Also, it describes the method of serving, consuming, and the manners to be followed during and after mealtime; it directs that ghee is to be served in black metal vessels, drinks in silver vessels, fruits on leaves, dry and sticky items in gold vessels, hard pieces in stoneware, drinking water in copper vessels, wines in glass or earthenware, and beverages in vessels studded with precious stones. The position to be allotted for each item is also specified. In the *Sūtrasthāna*, 46 chapters are devoted to these matters.

There are 16 chapters in the *Nidānasthāna*. This section discusses the aetiology of diseases that come under the purview of surgery. The first chapter is devoted to diseases caused by *vayu*, as it controls the functioning of the body. Further, it proceeds to the aetiology of diseases such as piles and calculus. Also, this part deals with diseases such as *sūka* and *upadamśa*. In those days, aphrodisiacs were in use, and their ill-effects caused suka and upadamśa, according to Suśruta, which are different from the veneral diseases of today.

There are 10 chapters in the *Śārīrasthāna*. The first deals with creation. This corresponds to the principles of the *sāṅkhya* system. Other theories that were then current, such as *svabhāvavāda*, *īsvaravāda*, *kālavāda*, *yadrcchāvāda*, *niyativāda*, and *pariṇāmavāda*, are also described. The subsequent chapters explain semen, blood, and the conception and development of the foetus. It states that the total number of bones in the human body is 103; the Vedic view accepted by Yājñavalkya and Agniveśa is also given in this part. Suśruta mentions that the basis of human nature is the three *doṣas*; the view of some *ācāryas* that it was based on the five principles (*mahābhūtas*) is also given. The tenth chapter is on paediatrics, which describes the labour room, equipment needed there, expectant mother's preferences and dislikes, the care for the baby, and so forth. It prescribes that the first food given to a child should be gold ground to a paste mixed with honey. This is prescribed in the *smrtis* and *Kāśyapasamhita* too. Naming the newborn is advised to be done on the 10th day. Since there was the belief of the affliction by evil spirits in Suśruta's time, he describes the methods to protect the child from them. He is of the view that the ideal age for sexual union for the female is above 16 and the above 25 for the male.

There are 40 chapters in the *Cikitsasthāna*; the first 23 chapters deal with surgical cases and their treatments. As ailments are of two kinds, wounds are also of two kinds—natural and accidental. Suśruta mentions 60 types of medical treatments for injuries (in Caraka, it is 36) and 6 types of sudden injuries (*sadyovraṇas*). In the treatment for broken bones (*bhagnacikitsa*), after bandaging bone joints, anointing with medicated oils, irrigation with medicated liquids, and so forth are prescribed. The procedure of surgery for piles and calculus is described in detail. Treatments for leprosy, diabetes, diabetic carbuncles, surgery for stomach disorders, inactive labour, and so forth are also explained in this chapter. Salt is not permitted for use after abdominal surgery; milk is prescribed for six months.

The next chapter on the maintenance of good health prescribes the *svasthavṛtta* and *sadvṛtta* (the code of conduct for ideal life). It is followed by rejuvenation and aphrodisiac therapies; details of changes that may occur in the body after different *rasāyana* therapies are also expressed. Details about oleation (*snēhana*), sweating (*svēdana*), emesis (*vamana*), purging (*virēcana*), and nine methods of oral cleaning (*gaṇḍūṣavidhi*) are given in the subsequent chapters.

There are eight chapters in the *Kalpasthāna*, which include toxicology. It discusses how the kings are being poisoned by enemies through food, garlands, and clothes during war, and the methods to combat it. Suśruta classifies poison into two groups, those of plant origin (*sthāvaraviṣa*) and those of animal origin (*jaṅgamaviṣa*), and studies their symptoms and treatments separately. In *sthāvaraviṣa*, he explains the different parts of the plant having toxicity; their symptoms and differences are also explained in detail. In *jaṅgamaviṣa*, the distinction between the serpents, the characteristics of their fang marks, their vengeance, and so on are explained. Apart from snakes, the symptoms and treatments for the poison of scorpions, tarantulas, spiders, and so forth are described. In one chapter, there are certain formulations that describe methods such as beating the drum smeared with medicated paste to purify the air. Then, it studies the poisons of rodents and rabies; in the chapter on *kīṭakalpa*, the symptoms and treatment for a wasp bite and so on are mentioned.

Thus, the five branches of Āyurveda, that is, surgery (*śalya*), paediatrics (*kaumārabhṛtya*), rejuvenation (*rasāyana*), aphrodisiacs (*vājīkaraṇa*), and healthy living (*svāstha*) are described in 120 chapters; another three branches, that is, ailments of organs such as the eyes, nose, ears, and head (*śālākya*), general medicine (*kāyacikitsa*), and demonology (*bhūtavidya*) are discussed in the *Uttaratantra*.

Uttaratantra

The *Uttaratantra* deals with the technique of surgical treatment for the removal of cataract. Here it may be noted in particular that Buddhist literature refers to Sribuddha as a surgeon who extracted the four poisoned arrows that pierced into the human body, namely anger, greed, pride, and jealousy. According to a recent scholar, this metaphor gave rise to numerous allusions to surgery in the Buddhist canonical texts: 'Thathagatha surpasses mundane physicians in Ophthalmology because he knows how to cut off *timira*, cataract, of ignorance with the tool of knowledge.[5] According to the same authority, this is an idea expressed in the *Samyuktagama*, attributed to the period of the Jin dynasty of the period 350–431 CE. She further mentions that such references to cataract surgery are many in the early Buddhist texts that were translated from the original Buddhist canonical texts into Chinese. If we go by the dates mentioned by Deshpande for the transmission of knowledge of cataract surgery to

[5] Vijaya Deshpande, 'Indian Influence on Early Chinese Ophthalmology: Glaucoma as a Case Study', *Bulletin of the School of Oriental and African Studies*, 1999, 62(2): 306–22.

China, it seems to suggest in unequivocal terms that cataract surgery was known to the surgeons prior to the composition of the *Uttaratantra* or that the dates of the composition of the text had to be pushed back in time prior to the date of the composition of that text, that is, earlier than the fourth century CE. Anyway, the Buddhist version comes from a popular version oft-quoted in the Brahminical texts as a mantra of the veneration to the guru.

There are 66 chapters in the *Uttaratantra*, which is appended to the Samhita. Apart from the description of ailments of the eyes, nose, ears, and head (*śālākya*), this portion explains demonology (*grahabādha*) of children and their treatments, the omitted portions of *kāyacikitsa*, and concludes with a description of *tantrayukti*. *Suśrutasamhita* also describes the then prevalent system of education, holidays, and so forth; the prescriptions strictly follow the scriptures. There are some interesting commands on methods of learning such as: one should learn science directly from a preceptor; practice should be only after sufficient training; learning should not be too fast nor intermittent; speech should be clear—not nasal or half-pronounced; during the period of study, the limbs should not dangle or the organs allowed to move; the voice should be refined and sweet; the seat should not be too high or too low; no one should interrupt the preceptor and disciple during lessons.

Suśruta emphasizes the need of interdisciplinary learning directly from the experts of each discipline and he points out that one must be humble enough and liberal to learn. Suśruta asserts that knowledge without understanding is just like the sandalwood carried by the donkey; seldom does it enjoy the fragrance! The scattered references in the text give us a picture of the customs and practices of that age. It also tells us about the high standard that medical science had attained by that time.

Rhinoplasty

Some scholars are of the opinion that the *Uttaratantra* is an addition to the original Samhita at a later epoch of history, most probably in the post-Gupta period. It has also been observed by some recent researchers that this portion is more technical than the rest of the portions in the Samhita.[6] This portion is historically important in that it

[6] Deshpande, 'Indian Influence on Early Chinese Ophthalmology', 306–22.

has some close connection with certain areas of sociopolitical formations in the subcontinent. Thus, Kautalya's *Arthaśāstra* informs us that the mutilation of the nose was a punishment given to some crimes, including killing of certain animals, abetment in theft, and adultery. Again, according to the *Manusmṛti*, 10 places on the human body where punishment for offences are to be inflicted in the case of non-Brahmins include the nose, in addition to the eyes, ears, hands, tongue, and so forth. Coming to later periods, during the Mughal and Sultanate eras, the mutilation of nose continued as a form of punishment. Surgeons of rhinoplasty and their methods of operation are also heard of from that period. When Akbar conquered the hill state of Kangra, the emperor was told that the place was widely known for four things: manufacturing of new noses, treatment of eye, basmati rice, and strong forts.[7] The *Suśrutasamhita* in general and the section on *śālākyatantra* in particular acquire added relevance and importance against these historical facts about the ancient Indian tradition of jurisprudence at least from the time of the Mauryan rule. Further, it may not be improbable to assume that the techniques, including the surgical treatments of rhinoplasty, were originally conceived and continued and developed in the later periods in order to cater to some contemporary social needs.

Training in Surgery

Suśruta, who is rightly qualified as a colossus of surgery, laid great emphasis on the training of surgeons. He maintains that a physician having textual knowledge without practical training is like a coward in the battlefield. Similarly, a bold and dexterous man lacking in textual knowledge would fail to succeed in his profession. A physician with half knowledge is like a bird with one wing.

One of the essential qualities of a surgeon is thorough knowledge of the human body. This has to be acquired by careful dissection and observation of the dead body (*Suśrutasamhita*: *Śārīrasthāna*, 5: 47–51). The body for dissection should be of a man who is not very old or wasted or chronically ill. He should not have been dead due to

[7] Susmita Basu Majumdar and Nayana Sharma Mukherjee, 'Two Nineteenth-Century Plastic Surgeons in India', in their *Essays on History of Medicine*, 58–9.

poisoning. The dead body should be put inside a cage, after covering with Muñja grass or Rusha or Sana. The cage is left submerged in a flowing stream in a dark place. After decaying for a week, it has to be taken out and rubbed with a brush of hair or bamboo. Then the soft portions are to be peeled off for careful observation of the structure of the body and the parts thereof. It is clear from this instruction that the method of acquisition of the knowledge of anatomy had already been systematized at the time of this text.

Practical Training

Practical training in the actual techniques of surgery is essential for students by the imaginative use of models of experiments. The basic procedures, as we have noted earlier, are *chedya* (excision), *bhēdya* (incision), *vēdhya* (puncturing), *ēśya* (probing), *āharya* (extraction), *visrāvya* (drainage), *sīvya* (suturing), *bandhana* (bandaging), *kṣāra* (alkali), *agni* (cautery), and *karnasandhibandha* (joining earlobes). For various acts of operation, things such as *kūśmāṇḍa* (*Benincasa hisbida*), jackfruit, alabu, urinary bladder of dead animals filled with slush, lotus stalk, bamboo pipes, teeth of dead animals, and so on are used. As mentioned earlier, it was compulsory to obtain permission from ruling authorities to practise surgery.

Surgical procedure: Pre- and post-operative care for patients is emphatically mentioned by Suśruta for a successful surgical operation. Surgical instruments and accessories should be ready for use. Apart from all these, strong attendants who are bold and friendly must be ready to help the surgeon. Prior to the operation, the patient and the relatives are to be informed about the acute necessity of the surgery. Patients are to be kept fasting before surgery. Needless to say, the premises, that is, the operation theatre, should be neat and clean, and free from dust and wind. Suśruta says that an auspicious time has to be fixed for the surgical intervention on the basis of astral position and so forth. Chanting of hymns suitable for the occasion is also suggested. Such measures point to the Brahminical connection with the treatment of patients. However, these were probably at a later date. Post-operative care included changing the dressings and bandages according to the season, and treatment for wounds. It is mentioned that the physician should act as a protective father to the patient.

It may not be out of place here to commit to memory the major contributions of this great Indian *ācārya* of surgical treatments under the tutelage of Āyurveda. The description of the method of dissecting dead bodies appears for the first time in Suśruta and on this issue he is often described as the 'Father of Anatomy' in the sense that he was responsible for the systematization of the topic in the scientific method. Skin, bones, joints, muscles, blood vessels, and so forth are described in the *Suśrutasamhita* in great detail. The importance of a practical knowledge of anatomy was considered essential by Suśruta for a successful surgeon.

Second, eight types of surgical operations were systematically arranged, which include all surgical treatments. Cesarean, section, lapratomy, and anorectal surgery are all described in the *Suśrutasamhita* in great detail. The book also describes 60 modes of treatment of wounds and ulcers along with various types of bandages. In addition to this, ancillary methods, such as *raktamokṣa* (blood-letting), cauterization, and application of caustic, were developed as a separate discipline under the name *kṣāratantra*. Urgent treatment for burns was also systematized by Suśruta.

Third, it was Suśruta who prescribed an effective methodology for imparting training in surgery by lectures, demonstrations, and practical studies in a systematic way. He designed various types of surgical instruments and implements in the shape of various animals, birds, and other creatures according to their specific needs on the operation table. These are named after the names of the corresponding species.

Plastic surgery, now an important branch of surgical operations, is considered to be the unique contribution of Suśruta. Taking into consideration all these achievements, Suśruta is rightly called the 'Father of Surgery'. Military medicine, a corollary of the subject of surgery, has its proper place in the *Suśrutasamhita*. Suśruta systematized the branch of toxicology and he provided it a status of science by classifying poisonous substances and prescribed suitable treatment for each of them. Above all these in the area of surgical operations, Suśruta developed some theoretical base for understanding diseases. For example, he identified five types of *pitta* and prescribed treatment for each of them.

In the field of fundamentals, Suśruta advanced the concepts. He traced the process of intrinsic pathology in the form of six *kriyākālas* and also drew the attention of physicians to the pathogenic importance of blood. His definition of *svasthavṛtta* remains the ideal one even today. Suśruta's contributions are remarkable in the field of drug science too. He advanced some of the concepts of pharmacopoeia and introduced many specific drugs. He classified the drugs into 37 *gaṇas* according to the therapeutic uses of them, with one *gaṇa* for mineral drugs.

It may not be irrelevant in this context to compare Western classical medicine and its practice in the field of surgical operations. In Greek and Roman antiquity, physicians turned to surgery only when drugs were not available. Hippocrates figures prominently in the history of Greek works on medicine and surgery in general, though all works in this category need not be taken to have been written by a single individual. The author of one such work entitled *On the Surgery* says that surgeons should know how they should proceed with treatment. Much of the work pertains to the work of bandaging various types of injuries. Hippocrates wrote around 400 BCE that the things related to surgery are the patient, the operator, the assistants, the instruments, the light, the time, the place, and the manner.

By the thirteenth and fourteenth centuries, surgery was denigrated and avoided by physicians who had received their education in the universities that were rising all over Europe. Medicine was usually one of the basic subjects of study. Surgeons, on the other hand, very often came from the unlettered lower classes and were scorned in clerical circles. Surgeons were taught the ways of their craft by apprenticeships.[8]

[8] Brieger, 'The Development of Surgery', 1–4.

5

Samhitas of Bhēḷa, Haritha, and Kasyapa, and Other Samhitas

Kāśyapasamhita

There are two or three texts with the same name, the *Kāśyapasamhita*. The one that is supposed to be 'the original' is obtained in a mutilated form in which the preface, conclusion, and some other parts are missing. The major theme of this work is *kaumārabhṛtya*, paediatrics. Another manuscript preserved in the Tanjavur library (no. 10780) is in the form of a discussion between Uma and Mahesvara. This was published only recently along with another text, *Jvarasamuccaya*. *Kaumārabhṛtya* is not the theme of this work. The style of composition is also different. Interestingly enough, some tantric procedures are mentioned. Scholars are of the opinion that this could be a modern work by another Kāśyapa.[1] A third text obtained from Chennai has preventive medicines as its central theme. Thus, we have at

[1] Varier, *History of Āyurveda*, 119–20.

least three texts with the same name. However, identifying the original work is not very difficult thanks to the style of composition and the nature of content.

The identity of Kāśyapa is, as usual, uncertain. There are certain names of clans, such as Kāśyapa, Bhrgu, Vasishta, and so forth, which on certain occasions meant not an individual but the clan as a whole. Here we do not know whether the nomenclature denotes a person or the clan to which he belonged. According to a story in the *Kalpasthāna* of *Kāśyapasamhita*, the *ācārya* Kāśyapa learnt the science through penance with the help of Brahma. He then imparted it to Jīvaka, the young son of Ricika. He learnt this science and compiled it. Being so young, other sages ridiculed this work as the prattle of a young boy. Humiliated by this, Jīvaka immersed himself in the Ganga at Kanakhal and came up as an aged man. The sages assembled there respectfully and called him 'Vṛdhajīvaka'. This text compiled by Jīvaka was lost and Anayasa, a *yakṣa,* recovered it. Later, Vatsya, a great scholar, redacted it and added the *Khilasthāna*. The text is also known as *Vṛdhajīvakīyatantra.* Even in this *Vṛdhajīvakīyatantra,* some portions are missing.

Interestingly, the available text of the *Kāśyapasamhita* adheres to the Vedic lore in the content as well as the style of composition. Offerings to Vedic deities such as Agni, Soma, and Prajāpati are mentioned. On the basis of these portions, N.V.K. Varier reasonably suggests that the text was composed in a period when Vedic rituals were popular in practice.[2] Atrideva Vidyalankar says that this work was compiled during the Gupta period. The *Kāśyapasamhita* contains the *mahā-mayūri* and other mantras that were prevalent in the period of Mahāyāna.

Kaumārabhṛtya is the subject matter of this work just as Suśruta deals with surgery. However, this need not necessarily mean that specialization of any kind was in vogue. Though the work focuses on paediatrics, the text deals with some other subjects also and some common diseases, such as acidity, different types of fever, and so forth. Demonology and *grahacikitsa* (treatment of illness caused by attack of demons) based on chants and sacrifices are also found in the text. This is called *Atharvana vidya.* In short, it may be concluded that the work betrays signs of a scientific text and at the same time it

[2] Varier, *History of Āyurveda,* 119–20.

contains some popular folk practices, such as magic and religious healing too. Perhaps this signifies an Indian trait of departure from the existing practice.

Bhēḷasamhita

Bhēḷa, also a legendary teacher and the celebrated author of *Bhēḷasamhita*, is believed to be one of the disciples of the great preceptor Ātreya and a colleague of Agniveśa. Pieces of information available on Bhēḷa, though incomplete, are quite interesting. Vāgbhaṭa, the author of *Aṣṭāṅgahṛdaya*, in order to corroborate the authority of his work, says in a critical view that the *Bhēḷasamhita*, even though composed by a sage, failed to get acceptance due to its poor construction.[3] Though this allegation, on the face of it in Vāgbhaṭa's time, is factual, it creates complications for researchers. The original text of this Samhita is believed to have been lost almost irrecoverably and there are several works that claim their origin to this work. That the *ācārya* was a predecessor to Vāghbhaṭa is clear since he is quoted by Vāgbhaṭa on several occasions.

A genius in medicine, Bhēḷa had his own knowledge about human nature. He developed some novel ideas about the position of the mind in the human body. It is important to note that Bhēḷa's knowledge of the 'mind' is different from the notion of the same of Caraka and Suśruta. He is perhaps more precise in presupposing that the human mind is situated between the upper palate and the brain, whereas according to Caraka and Suśruta it is in the heart (*hṛdaya*). This hypothetic idea is taken by some scholars to indicate some pre-Vedic wisdom. According to some recent scholars, Bhēḷa inherited the ideals of the Indus civilization, while Caraka and Suśruta followed the knowledge of the Vedic age.[4] Though Bhēḷa and Agniveśa learnt the science of Āyurveda from the same preceptor, the difference of opinion about such concepts provides the opportunity to a critical evaluation by the present generations of researchers in Āyurveda.

[3] M.S. Valiathan, *The Legacy of Vāgbhaṭa* (Hyderabad: University Press, 2013), xvi.

[4] See Varier, *History of Āyurveda*, 78.

Bhēḷa's Study of the Mind

Bhēḷa's study of the mind differed from that of Caraka and Suśruta. Bhēḷa and Agniveśa studied under the same preceptor; then how do they differ? In fact, one must have had a clear idea about the seat of the brain even in the period of the Samhitas. From the primitive period, man, who lived by hunting, had occasions to learn that the head was the centre of all movements; the scenes of partially or completely damaged heads of animals might have been the source of this learning. Egypt, Greece, and India had this knowledge from very ancient times. The *yogamudras* (yogic postures) recovered from the Indus Valley excavations show the development of yoga; *yogaśāstra* shows the head as the centre of intelligence, the sense organs, and the mind. So, there is no wonder that Bhēḷa knew this, but the slip-up that occurred in Caraka and Suśruta is strange. Gananathsen Sarasvati in his 'Introduction' to *Pratyakṣaśārīra* points out errors that have crept into the study of anatomy in later times. Several instances can be seen in ancient works where corruptions and interpolations have been made at the hands of their redactors and teachers.

A reference has already been made to two streams of thought in India: successors to the Indus Valley civilization who, according to experts, had knowledge about physiology, and the Vedic tradition, which emphasized the use of medicine accompanied by the chanting of hymns.[5] The outlook of both must have changed after the period of the Samhitas. Usually, the works that one prefers to study and popularize would be in line with the prevalent ideology, and thus Āyurveda must have been modified to suit the philosophy of the Vedic people. The people who handled *Bhēḷasamhita* might have been under the influence of the Indus Valley civilization. Or else, the prominence achieved by Caraka and Suśruta at the time of the Vedic tradition might have been denied to Bhēḷa. Vāgbhaṭa refers to the elegant style of Caraka and Suśruta. They must have achieved this elegance by their magnificent redaction. The Samhitas that were current in Vāgbhaṭa's time had undergone much redaction and updating. The indifference of the Vedic people for tantrism must also be reckoned with. Be that as it may, Bhēḷa was a preceptor, acceptable to the followers of all systems. All the *ācāryas* consider his views and formulations as authentic.

[5] See Varier, *History of Āyurveda*, 20–1.

Hārītasamhita

Hārīta is considered to be one of the disciples of Ātreya and a contemporary of Agniveśa. The available text consists of six *sthānas*. The first *sthāna* describes basic principles, seasonal regime, and constitution of the human body; *dravyaguṇa*, medicinal properties of various herbs, and other substances, including urine; different types of grains, grams, leaves, fruits, honey, meat; and so forth. The second *sthāna* deals with the different types of diseases, their aetiology and treatments, psychiatric problems, and so forth. The third *sthāna* deals with the problems of sleep and *riṣṭalakṣaṅa* (signs of ailment). The fourth *sthāna* mentions the systems of measurements, mode of preparation of medicated oils, sudation therapy, *vasti* (enema), and *raktamokṣa* (blood-letting). The fifth *sthāna* contains different medicinal fruits, such as *harītaki, triphala, rasona*, and so forth. The sixth *sthāna* deals with the subjects of anatomy and physiology.

1. *Sthāna* I: 23 chapters
2. *Sthāna* II: 9 chapters
3. *Sthāna* III: 58 chapters
4. *Sthāna* IV: 6 chapters
5. *Sthāna* V: 5 chapters
6. *Sthāna* VI: 1 chapter

What appears to be evident from the traditions of these Samhitas and their authors is that the knowledge of Āyurveda was systematized in the age of these treatises. These works show that the art of healing and healthcare, coming from a hoary past, had attained the form of a science with a definite method of compilation, preservation, and transmission.

Vāgbhaṭa

Vāgbhaṭa, also known as Vāhaṭa, is the celebrated physician and the author of *Aṣṭāṅgahṛdaya* and *Aṣṭāṅgasaṅgraha*. Biographical information, date, and other details of Vāgbhaṭa are extremely scanty. In such a situation, it is better to listen to the author himself. The *Aṣṭāṅgasaṅgraha* concludes with a verse that states that the text was composed by a learned physician named Vāgbhaṭa. According to the same verse, the author's grandfather was also named Vāgbhaṭa and he too was a great physician. The author was the son of Simhagupta, a physician and the son of the senior Vāgbhaṭa. Thus, we get a lineage of three physicians. The author of the *Aṣṭāṅgasaṅgraha* says that he was born in Sindhudesa and that his preceptor was Avalokita. Vāgbhaṭa learnt the science of Āyurveda from this Avalokita and his father Simhagupta. These are the facts available about Vāgbhaṭa and with this the scholars have created all sorts of controversies and debates regarding the authorship of the two popular texts of the science of Āyurveda. Unfortunately, the author Vāgbhaṭa is silent about his date, the important events of his lifetime, and of his contemporaries, which has also provided a lacuna for the scholars to make all sorts of speculations.

Aṣṭāṅgahṛdaya started attracting scholarly attention from within the country and abroad within a short period of its composition. Commentaries for this celebrated text started appearing from that early date. The earlier commentators include the famous scholars of the subject, such as Aruṇadatta, Bhaṭṭa, Narahari, Candra, Indu, and so forth. The text was translated into the Tibetan language with the title *Rgud Bzi* during the years 755 to 797 CE. A translation in Arabic was brought out during the reign of the well-known Khalifa Harun Al Rashid, the celebrated character of the *Arabian Nights* (773 to 808 CE). *Aṣṭāṅgahṛdaya* is cited as one of the major works in Āyurveda by a Persian physician, the author of *Firdaus Al-Hikma* in 850 CE.[6] It may be safely assumed on the basis of this information that Vāgbhaṭa belonged to a period earlier than the eighth century BCE.

Both the *Aṣṭāṅgasaṅgraha* and *Aṣṭāṅgahṛdaya* follow closely the teaching of the great *ācāryas*, including Caraka, Suśruta, and so forth, and acknowledge their authority of him in the portion *kāyacikitsa*. At the same time, what is historically significant is the evolution of the knowledge of Āyurveda in terms of its philosophical backgrounds. A distinctive departure is clear in both the *Aṣṭāṅgasaṅgraha* and the *Aṣṭāṅgahṛdaya* from Caraka in the basic concept of *pañcabhūta*, the five basic elements of earth, water, fire, wind, and ether. It has been observed that the *Aṣṭāṅgasaṅgraha* and *Aṣṭāṅgahṛdaya* skipped off such associated questions also, such as the relation between *prakṛti* and *purusha* (human microcosm), the homology between the human microcosm

[6] Zysk, *Asceticism and Healing in Ancient India.*

and the universal macrocosm, the relation between the body and its knower, and so forth.[7] Similarly, Caraka dwells at length on the basis of the theories of the Vaiśeṣika system of philosophy, on concepts such as guṇa, that is, quality inherent in substances. These are also left untouched by Vāgbhaṭa. He is more inclined towards the practical and down-to-earth details of diseases and treatments. The same trend is visible in customs, such as the intiation ceremony of the students and the oath to be administered by the preceptor, condemnations of quacks and imposters, and so forth. A notable change seems to have occurred in relation to the number and composition of medicinal formulations, which showed no decrease in the *Aṣṭāṅgasaṅgraha*, but in the *Aṣṭāṅgahṛdaya* the number seems to decline.

At the same time, continuity can be traced in the case of the idea of causal connections of the diseases, stipulation of 11 major clinical features, eligibility on the basis of good health, and so forth. The role of evacuative therapy has not changed significantly from the Samhita to the *Aṣṭāṅgasaṅgraha* or *Aṣṭāṅgahṛdaya*.

Aṣṭāṅgahṛdaya

The work is an abridged version of the *Aṣṭāṅgasaṅgraha.*[8] It is also an improvement on the original work. The *Aṣṭāṅgahṛdaya* consists of the core substance of the teachings of the earlier authorities, including Caraka, Suśruta, Bhēḷa, Hārīta, and so forth. The text is noted for its literary quality and crisp and apt presentation. The text contains 6 sections and 120 chapters in about 7,120 verses. Different texts are available and they vary in the number of verses, thereby implying that omissions and additions were made from time to time. The *Aṣṭāṅgahṛdaya* is perhaps a text that has the highest number of commentaries when compared to the other classics, such as the Samhitas of Caraka and Suśruta. The most famous commentary of the *Aṣṭāṅgahṛdaya* is *Sarvāṅgasundari*. The historical importance of the *Aṣṭāṅgahṛdaya* lies in the fact that it is an improved and developed form of an earlier text the *Aṣṭāṅgasaṅgraha*. The *Aṣṭāṅgasaṅgraha* is composed with a mixture of prose and verse in an archaic style of composition, whereas the *Aṣṭāṅgahṛdaya* is composed in verse alone.

[7] Valiathan, *The Legacy of Vāgbhaṭa*, xvi.

[8] Valiathan, *The Legacy of Vāgbhaṭa*, xvi.

The versified form of the text goes a long way in helping students and practitioners of the sciences in memorizing the same.

Significantly enough, the *Aṣṭāṅgahṛdaya* shows a peculiarity in its treatment of the subject. The author has omitted several of the religious rituals as well as social customs and practices referred to in the original *Aṣṭāṅgasaṅgraha*. The *Aṣṭāṅgahṛdaya* perhaps has the largest number of commentaries rather than the classical Samhitas of Caraka and Suśruta. No wonder the *Aṣṭāṅgahṛdaya* is included in the 'Great Triad (*Bṛhtrayi*) of Āyurveda'.

Aṣṭāṅga Ayurveda has eight branches. They are:

1. *Kāya*, general medicine
2. *Bāla*, paediatrics
3. *Graha*, demonology or psychiatric treatment
4. *Ūrdhvāṅga*, head and the upper limbs
5. *Śalya*, surgery
6. *Damṣṭra*, toxicology
7. *Jara*, geriatrics
8. *Vṛṣa*, enhancement of sexual potency

Kāyacikitsa deals with systemic illnesses, that is, the diseases arising from disorders of digestive activity, known in modern parlance as inner medicine. *Bālacikitsa* is the treatment of diseases of children (paediatrics), *grahacikitsa* denotes the treatment of diseases from being possessed by evil sprits, pathogenic micro-organisms, and so forth, and deals mainly with mental diseases (psychiatry). *Ūrdhvāṅgacikitsa* deals with the treatment of diseases of the head, including the eyes (ophthalmology), ears (otology), nose (rhinology), throat (laryngology), and teeth (dentistry). *Śalyacikitsa*, also known as *Śastracikitsa*, deals with the treatments requiring the use of knife (surgery). *Damṣṭracikitsa* means the treatment of diseases due to poison (toxicology). *Jaracikitsa*, also known as *rasāyanacikitsa*, deals with the treatment of diseases of old age (geriontology, geriatrics). *Vṛṣacikitsa* deals with the treatment of diseases such as impotency, sterility, and so forth, and making man sexually virile by the use of aphrodisiacs.

Nature and contents of the *Aṣṭāṅgahṛdaya*

The *Aṣṭāṅgahṛdaya* contains 6 *sthānas*, each *sthāna* consisting of varying number of *adhyāyas*, chapters, the total number of chapters being 120. The text is composed entirely in verse. The total number of verses is 7,120 in the extant edition.[9] In addition, there are about 33 verses that have not been commented upon by Aruṇadatta, hence considered as later interpolations. There are 240 short prose lines too, 2 at the commencement of each chapter. The *sthānas* and their important contents are given below:

1. *Sūtrasthāna*: 30 chapters
2. *Śārīrasthāna*: 6 chapters
3. *Nidānasthāna*: 16 chapters
4. *Cikitsasthāna*: 22 chapters
5. *Kalpasthāna*: 6 chapters
6. *Uttarasthāna*: 40 chapters

Sūtrasthāna, the first section, has 30 chapters dealing with basic doctrines of Āyurveda, principles of health, prevention of diseases, property of articles of diet and drugs, humoral physiology and pathology, different kinds of diseases, and methods of treatment. It describes the basic doctrines and principles of healthy prevention of diseases, diet, food habits, causes of diseases, methods of treatment, and so forth.

Śārīrasthāna, the second section, has six chapters dealing with the topics of the evolution of the universe, embryology, anatomy, physiology, physiognomy, physical and psychological constitutions, auspicious and inauspicious dreams and omens, signs of bad prognosis, and of oncoming death. It is worth noting in this connection that here the mind is considered to be part of the body.

Nidānasthāna, the third section, with 16 chapters describes the causes, premonitory symptoms, characteristic features, pathogenesis, and prognosis of some important diseases coming within the realm of *kāyacikitsa* (general inner medicine).

Cikitsasthāna, the fourth section, has 22 chapters elaborating the methods of treatment of all major organic diseases pertaining to the topic of *Kāyacikitsa*, including therapeutic strategies, efficacious medicinal recipes, diet, and care of the patient.

[9] Harisastry Paradhkar, ed., *Aṣṭāṅgahṛdaya* (Bombay: Nirnayasagar Press, 1939; reprinted Varanasi: Chaukhambha Orentalia, 1982).

Kalpasthāna, the fifth section, has six chapters dealing with the preparation of recipes, strategies of purgative treatment (*pañcakarma*), administration of purificatory therapies, and management of complications; as well as the principles of pharmacy weights and measures, and the allied subjects.

Uttarasthāna, the sixth and the last section, is devoted to the remaining 7 branches of Āyurveda. It has 40 chapters in total; divided as follows, 3 for *bālacikitsa* (paediatrics), 4 for *grahacikitsa* (psychiatry or, as it is incorrectly translated, demonology), 17 for *ūrdhvāṅgacikitsa* (diseases of upper organs in the head)—subdivided again: 9 for *netracikitsa* (ophthalmology), 2 for *karṇacikitsa* (otology), 2 for *nāsācikitsa* (rhinology), 2 for *mukhacikitsa* (mouth, teeth, and throat), and 2 for *siroroga* (diseases of the head)—*śalyacikitsa* (surgery) has 10 chapters; *damṣṭra* (toxicology) has 4; and *jarācikitsa* (or *rasāyana*, which includes rejuvenation therapy, geriatrics, and so on) and *vṛṣa* (or *vājīkaraṇa*, which includes virilizing therapy, aphorodisiacs, and so on) have 1 chapter each.

6

Ancient Indian Medical Education

Ancient Indian medicine and its practice find mention in Vedic hymns, which are the earliest of the Indian literary sources. According to these hymns, the healing practices are associated with the *bhiṣak* who is described as *kavi*, an expert in the recitation of the hymns; and *vipra*, literally meaning 'shaker' and performer of the ritual in the present Vedic context. These literary references appear to imply that the *bhiṣaks* are the custodians of a specialized knowledge of healing and healthcare. What seems to follow is that the strategies of healing require some form of learning. Scholars of Vedic literature such as J. Gonda have convincingly shown that the techniques of composition and recitation of Vedic hymns are oral formulaic in nature.[1] Against this background, it can be reasonably assumed that the learning of the chanting of hymns and the performance of rituals were on the basis of memorization of the formulaic elements during the Vedic period. This necessitated repeated recitation, memorizing, and performance. In all probability, this is the earliest form of medical education in ancient

[1] J. Gonda, *Vedic Literature* (Weisbaden: Otto Harrassowitz, 1975), 23–4.

India. According to the *Dharmaśāstra* of a later date, *bhiṣaks*, who were the custodians of the knowledge of medicine, enjoyed a lower status in society, probably for the reason that they often moved with all sections in society, including foreign groups, for various purposes such as acquisition of medical knowledge. An acute paucity of sources, however, prevents us from making any comments regarding the details of this early form of training.

The knowledge of medicine and its practice was reduced to writing for the first time in the Buddhist monasteries. The transition from orality to literacy presupposes a series of changes at deeper levels of the economy, society, and culture, but these are outside the ambit of this volume. Here, we only observe that the pressing need for the art of writing first occurred to the Vaiśya traders who were a section in society that provided support for heterodox sections, such as the Buddhists, Jains, Ājīvakas, and so forth. Among these, the early Buddhist *saṅgha* was engaged in providing medical care to the *bhikṣus* as well as to the lay worshippers following the advice of the Buddha himself. This necessitated some form of education and training for those who were involved in the management of diseases in the monastic institutions. Gradually, the *saṅgha* took the initiative in codifying the knowledge of medicine. This is perhaps the first stage in the institutionalization of ancient Indian medical education.

Takṣaśila, or Taxila, often described as a university, was perhaps one of the most famous and the highest seat of learning during the period under consideration. The place had already become prominent during the lifetime of the Buddha himself. Jīvaka Komārabhacca, a legendary character and celebrated physician who once treated Gautama Buddha himself, is said to have been educated at Taxila for seven years. Great Indian masters and *ācāryas* of medicine, such as Ātreya, Agniveśa, Bheḷa, Hārīta, and so forth, are associated with this high seat of learning, which set the standard for the universities in ancient India in their systems of teaching, learning, and examination. Some Jātaka stories relate the tale of how a *bōdhisattva* who studied at Taxila treated the king of Kāśi. Taxila remained a centre of excellence for several centuries until it was destroyed by the Huns who invaded India in the fifth century CE.

Towards the end of the Gupta dynasty, there was a resurgence of the old university tradition as noticed and described by the Chinese traveller Hsuan-tsang. He has given an excellent account of the Nālanda *mahāvihāra* (great *vihāra*) and the university. According to Hsuan-tsang, students came from distant places to Nālanda for higher studies in all subjects, including medicine, under great scholars.[2] The curriculum of study at the Nālanda University included all traditional subjects, such as Vedas, grammar, philology, logic, and so forth, in addition to the Mahāyāna texts. This seems to imply that the Brahminic attitude to the formal study of the Vedas and moving with other sections outside their caste had undergone considerable changes. *Cikitsa vidya* or medical education consisted mainly of the study of medicine, exorcism, use of stones and needles, and so forth. I-Tsing, another Chinese pilgrim, who visited India towards the end of the seventh century, mentions the five subjects of study, including medicine, and the eight parts thereof (*Aṣṭāṅga*).[3] Kenneth Zysk observes that 'medical knowledge by the middle of the seventh century was codified as a system that was preserved in the classical medical treatises and well established in the curriculum as one of the five sciences taught in the Buddhist Monastic universities'.[4]

Teaching and learning were properly systematized during the time of the Samhitas and this can be explicitly found in the *Carakasamhita* that lays specific rules and regulations at various stages of learning medicine. Caraka does not, however, mention Takṣaśila. It is assumed that side by side with the university stream of education, the ancient *gurukula* (teacher's residence) system also flourished for the training of physicians and that mode of teaching and learning attracted great masters as well as talented students. What can be learnt from the *Carakasamhita* is that the aspirant was obliged to have had sufficient learning in the formal subjects, such as grammar, logic, poetics, philosophy, and also astronomy, astrology, mathematics, botany, and so forth. Formal initiation to these traditional subjects would enable the aspirant to choose a particular text or branch of medical knowledge for detailed study. There was a rigorous process for the selection of a medical student. Physical, mental, and intellectual capacity as well as moral attributes were tested at the time of entry into the course of study. It may be noted that the teacher

[2] Zysk, *Asceticism and Healing in Ancient India*, 48.

[3] I-Tsing, *A Record of the Buddhist Religion as Practiced in India, and the Malayalam Archipelago*, trans. J. Takakusu (Delhi: Munshiram Manoharlal, 1982), 127–8.

[4] Zysk, *Asceticism and Healing in Ancient India*, 48.

accepted no more than a limited number of students at a time and each student received personal attention. At the time of initiation, the pupils had to undergo a formal procedure in which an oath was taken. According to the *Carakasamhita*, the ceremony was Vedic in character with the sacrificial fire, chanting of hymns, and oblation to the fire. In the Caraka tradition, the oath was taken at the commencement and not at the conclusion of the course of the training. The training of a physician had three components, namely, learning, instruction, and discussion. The textual *sutras* had to be learnt by rote. At the same time, the student was obliged to understand their meaning through long hours of study. The preceptor instructed the pupil on the textual passages and made sure that the students' pronunciation, intonation, and understanding were flawless. Debates and discussions were held in high esteem during the time of the study of medicine. Debates, both friendly and hostile, were prescribed, which helped the students equip themselves with the capacity to face any encounter in the future. This was, however, not restricted to medicine alone but prescribed for other subjects of study too.

Thorough textual and theoretical knowledge should be supported by an effective practical wisdom for an aspirant medical student in order to become a successful physician in the future. Suitable exercises are, therefore, prescribed with a view to equipping the pupils with necessary training in diagnosing the diseases and in prescribing the appropriate medicine. Effective exercises were given to enhance practical knowledge in the techniques of diagnostic methods, identification of herbs, preparation of various forms of medicines, and mastering therapeutic strategies. Special attention was paid for imparting training in surgical operations.[5]

Noble character and conduct are the most vital aspects of a physician, as envisioned by the great *ācāryas*. Emphasis is always on the principles of dharma, the supreme ideal of life according to the *Dharmaśāstras*. On the auspicious occasion of the beginning of the course of studies, the preceptor gave solemn advice to the pupil on these principles.

The *varṇa* system had its authority on all important walks of life and, quite naturally, it laid down instructions for learning medicine. However, Suśruta states that the knowledge of medicine may be

[5] See the chapter on 'Suśruta'.

imparted to all the four *varṇas*.[6] At the same time, the right to teach was restricted to the three upper sections, namely the Brāhmaṇa, the Kṣatriya, and the Vaiśya. While a Brahmin could give *dīkṣa* (formal advice) to the three upper sections, the Kṣatriya could teach a Kṣatriya, and a Vaiśya could teach a Vaiśya alone. Śūdras were imparted medical knowledge without the initiation ceremony.

Āyurveda beyond the Indian Subcontinent

The Buddhist *saṅgha* and its programmes of compassion were instrumental in the spread of the ancient Indian knowledge and practice of medicine to countries beyond the Indian subcontinent. Mahāyāna Buddhism and its medical and esoteric practices travelled as far as China via the Central Asian trade routes as early as the beginnings of the Common Era. Interestingly enough, the stories of the legendary character Jīvaka also became popular in China. In the Chinese language, he was called K'i-yu. It appears to be significant that the Bower manuscript, a Buddhist text in the Sanskrit language containing a large section on medicine, was discovered in Kuchar, an oasis and settlement in eastern Turkistan, situated on the caravan route to China.[7] Some parts of this manuscript are written in the Gupta Brāhmi characters of the fourth or fifth centuries CE. We learn from the Mahāyāna text, the *Saddharmapuṇḍarīka* in Sanskrit, that Bodhisatva Bhaiṣajyarājan became popular in the East Asian regions and attracted a large following of the Mahāyāna Buddhists. Zysk observes that the Buddhist monk healer Bhaiṣajyaguru became an object of worship in Central Asia and Kashmir around the third century CE, and in China by the next century.[8] Another evidence of connection between the Chinese treatment and the Indian system of medicine is available in the form of Chinese translations of Āyurvedic texts in Sanskrit. *Rāvaṇakumāratantra*, an Indian text dealing with pediatrics, is an example. Another example is a fragmented rendering of the *Kāśyaparṣiprokta Cikitsasūtra* into the Chinese language. Another text that is closely connected to the *Kāśyapasamhita* also found its way to the Chinese language.

6 Valiathan, *The Legacy of Suśruta*, 7.

7 Zysk, *Asceticism and Healing in Ancient India*, 62.

8 Zysk, *Asceticism and Healing in Ancient India*, 62–3.

Eye care as part of the *śālākya* (management of head and neck and their diseases) strategies was widely known in the Buddhist monasteries and in Āyurveda.[9] It is widely known that ancient Indian cataract surgery had won high reputation in the West as well as in the East. Indian therapeutic strategies of cataract were introduced to China as early as the medieval period, probably between the seventh and the ninth centuries.

Apart from the religious realm, there were contacts at the conceptual level as pointed out by some medical ideas of India and China. An example comes from the idea of the causation of disease.[10]

Esoteric practices of the Mahāyāna Buddhism, such as those included in the *Mantrayāna* and *Vajrayāna* traditions, became popular in Tibetan Buddhism. These practices consisted, among other things, of the learning of magical powers to cure diseases and also to ward off evil spirits and methods to prolong life. Buddhist monks and monk-healers were able to win followers who requested the services of monks in dealing with the extra-human forces. In short, magical healing practices became an integral part of Tibetan Buddhism. An important result of this spread of religious ideas and ideals was that the empirico-rational medicine of Āyurveda also was exported to these lands along with the magico-religious healing practices. In the Tibetan Buddhist canon, these were known as *Kanjur* and *Tanjur*.

Tibetan historian Bu-ston records that the *Aṣṭāṅgahṛdaya* was one of the principal texts followed in Tibet for the study of medicine. According to the same source, a translation of the work in the Tibetan language was available.[11] Zysk observes that 'by about the fourteenth century the curriculum involving the five sciences was an integral part of education in the Buddhist monasteries of Tibet'.[12]

[9] The theme of a Jātaka story and a Buddhist sculpture at Bharhut supports this early Indian achievement.

[10] Zysk, *Asceticism and Healing in Ancient India*, 65–6.

[11] Zysk, *Asceticism and Healing in Ancient India*, 48.

[12] Zysk, *Asceticism and Healing in Ancient India*, 62.

7

Regional Developments

We have seen that information about the advent in Tamiḻakam of the established tradition of medical treatment is in the edicts of the Mauryan emperor Ashoka. The Major Rock Edict II of Ashoka makes a categorical statement that he made arrangements for two kinds of treatments, that is, treatment for humans and that for animals (*manusacikicha ca pasucikicha*), in the territories of the Cōḻās, the Pāṇḍyas, and the Keralaputras.[1] Apart from the propagation of the Buddhist idea of compassion, this seems to imply that there was a demand for the fruits of such an imperial project of social welfare from the communities in the territories mentioned in the record. Tamil sources of the period between second century BCE and first century CE that were in the form of Tamil heroic songs have only scanty references to local traditions of healing and healthcare. A song in the *Purāṇaṉūṟu* alludes to *maruttuvamanai*, the residence of a medicine man.[2] Such evidences are inadequate for understanding the salient features of a tradition. Judging from the available sources, it can be assumed that the custodians of the art of healing in the far south were members of the community of Velans who were the traditional performers

[1] D.C. Sircar, *Asoka's Inscriptions* (Delhi: Publication Division, 1968).

[2] *Puṛānaṉūṛu*, 241.

of a particular rite called *veriyatal*. The healing practices of the Velans must have consisted of magical rites and other techniques of healing, including the use of medicines.

The system introduced by Ashoka was, in all probability, the one developed into a science in the Buddhist *vihāras* of the northern territories. Ashoka's interest in the Buddhist *saṅghas* and their programmes is too well known to call for any further explanation. It has been suggested on the basis of Pāli and Sanskrit sources that the shift of paradigm in the ancient Indian healing and healthcare system into an 'empirico-rational medicine' was an achievement of the ascetics in the Buddhist *vihāras*.[3] One or two points in this regard appear to be noteworthy in this cultural transaction. First, the local Tamil tradition came under the influence of a Prakrit tradition of heterodox groups. As a rule, the earliest phase of the science of Āyurveda is traced to the Vedic hymns mainly from the *Atharvaveda* and to a lesser extent from the *Ṛgveda*, which contain numerous references to a medicine lore mixed with myth, magic, and miracle. Here, in the Mauryan sources, the reference is to an instituted process of *cikīcha* (treatment). Second, and more importantly, the system introduced by the imperial strategy was, by nature, authentic and dominant due to its institutional base and theoretic acumen. Inscriptional sources of the subsequent period in various places in the southern parts of Tamiḻakam inform us that the Jaina ascetics and teachers in different parts of the Tamil south were engaged in imparting knowledge to the local students of medical science.[4] Significantly, the Tamil Āyurvedic texts, such as the *Ēlādi*, the *Jīvakcintāmaṇi nāṉmaṇikkōvai*, and the *Tirikaṭukam*, are attributed to this period. It may not be incorrect to assume that this was the first stage of a transition in the native non-classical tradition of healing and healthcare in ancient Tamiḻakam, including Kerala. A random examination of these texts goes to prove that the traces of a local tradition are not discernible in them and that they contain knowledge and information gathered from the Prakrit or Sanskrit texts of northern India. A logical conclusion would be that an indigenous system of medicine had not developed in Tamiḻakam in that distant past to be incorporated into the science coming from the northern parts of the subcontinent. However, we do not know to what extent the local

[3] Zysk, *Asceticism and Healing in Ancient India*, 21–2.

[4] R. Niranjana Devi, *Medicine in South India* (Chennai: Easwar Press, 2006), 186–7.

tradition of the Velans was influenced by the Buddhist scientific tradition coming from northern India.

The subsequent period witnessed a great transformation of society in the whole of South India, including Kerala. The earlier *ur* (settlements) and their *tiṇai* (traditional division of settlements) methods of production and distribution of resources gave way to the newly emerging agrarian villages. These new village settlements were 'near self-sufficient units' of economic production and reproduction as shown by the village studies.[5] Each village developed as a sustainable unit with all the necessary groups of artisans and craftsmen, such as carpenters, blacksmiths, goldsmiths, and other service groups, such as washermen, barbers, astrologers, medicine-men, midwives, and so on, in addition to the unskilled groups of tillers.[6] Burton Stein described the system as the 'localization of goods and services'.[7] It is important to note in the present context that the community of Velans with their traditional healing practices continued to flourish in Kerala in this period of agrarian villages, while their community disappeared altogether from the regions outside Kerala. The services of male members of the Velan community as medicine-men and performers of magico-religious rites and their womenfolk as village midwives were indispensable in the ensuing social life in all the settlements in Kerala throughout the medieval ages.

A distinctive stage in the history of Āyurveda is discernible in the innumerable village settlements in medieval Tamiḻakam and Kerala. The source material for understanding this development is in the form of inscriptions on stone and copper plates found in the Brahminical temples, mostly situated in the rural villages. These temples acted as community centres for all practical purposes during the period under discussion. Kenneth Zysk may be right in arguing that the Hindu temples at a later period made arrangements for providing

[5] M. N. Srinivas, ed., *India's Villages* (Delhi: Asia Publishing, 1960 [1955]), 40–55.

[6] For a detailed study of the villages in Tamil Nadu, see the chapter 'Village Community, Myth or Reality', in N. Karashima, *South Indian History and Society* (Delhi: Oxford University Press, 1984). For a detailed study of the villages in Kerala, see M.R. Raghava Varier, *Village Community in Pre-colonial Kerala* (Delhi: Asian Educational Services, 1994).

[7] Borton Stein (ed.), *Essays on South India* (Delhi: Vikas Publishing House, 1976).

medical services to the poor and the sick following the trend set by the Buddhist monastic institutions.[8] Whether adopting the Buddhist model or independently responding to the demands from the contemporary socio-economic set-up, it is a fact that Hindu temples in Tamil Nadu started figuring as centres of medical services at least from the early medieval period onwards. Significantly, as informed by contemporary epigraphic documents, there were also seats of learning attached to the Brahminical temples, thereby implying that the classical knowledge of medicine had rooted firmly in the religious culture of South India. It has to be noted in this connection that there is an attempt in the classical texts of Āyurveda to suppress the contributions of the Buddhists monasteries and the Pāli texts in accumulating empirico-rational ideas of diseases and medicine. The classical texts of Āyurveda are keen in assimilating this heterodox knowledge and wisdom of healthcare. At the same time, they are totally silent about the monastic phase of the indigenous traditions of healthcare. As part of this programme, the origin and early transmission of the knowledge of medicine is always traced to Hindu divinities, such as Indra, Brahma, and also to some great *ṛṣis* (saints). The earliest evidences for this spatial shift of medical services into the Hindu religious centres are the epigraphic records from the ninth century CE.

Champakalakshmi has convincingly shown that two major trends were working at deeper levels of the above-mentioned changes in the surface—decline of trade, both inland and maritime, and the emergence of land as the main resource. This is followed by a land grant system and an agrarian order, which brought in a hierarchically structured organization and a monarchical polity based on the principles of the *Dharmaśāstra*.[9] According to the same author, religious rivalry and persecution are closely related to the political patronage extended by the various dynasties of southern India. Hagiological works of the Bhakti movement, such as the *Periyapurāṇam*, contain stories of persecution of the heterodox sections, such as the Buddhists and Jains. These stories are to some extent corroborated by archaeological evidences in the form of dilapidated structural buildings. In Kerala, there are several Buddhist and Jaina sites that were transformed into Hindu shrines as in the cases of the Paḷḷibhagavathi Temple near Palakkad in

[8] Zysk, *Asceticism and Healing* in Ancient India, 46.

[9] Champakalakshmi, *Religion, Tradition and Ideology: Pre-Colonial South India* (Delhi: OUP, 2011), 438–9.

Malabar and also the Bharanikkavu Temple, south of Kottayam, and some idols in Mavelikkara and surrounding places. At the Paḷḷibhagavati Temple, the main deity Jvālāmālini Yakṣi, the protecting deity of Candraprabha, the eighth Tīrthaṅkara of Jains, became a *bhagavati* (female deity) of the Hindu pantheon. Candraprabha Tirthankara, who is enshrined in a small roofless structure, began to be worshipped as Śiva but the characteristic *lāñchanas* show the real identity of the idol.[10] These changes explain the early medieval developments in the area of medical services in South Indian villages.

The temples in medieval Tamil Nadu have yielded epigraphic documents containing information about medical services, including surgery. Information culled out from the epigraphic documents from the eighth to the thirteenth century CE supply interesting details about various aspects of Āyurvedic treatment in South India. The earliest of the documents mentions the names of some physicians who were holding high positions in the political level too. Thus, the *vaidyan* (physician) MāṛaṉKāri was the *uttaramantri* (chief minister) of the Pāṇḍyan king Māṛan Caṭaiyan who ruled towards the end of the eighth century CE. His brother Māṛan Eyia, also a member of that family of physicians, is stated to have followed his brother in the office of Māṛa Caṭaya.[11] Inscriptions from various temples in medieval Tamil Nadu mention the names of several such physicians as given below:

1. Aṅgavaidyan Kūttapperumān
2. Savarṇan Kulaśēkhara Nārāyaṇa of Kuḍanāḍu
3. Satrumāia Ālappirāntā
4. Savarṇan kōtaṇṭarāma of Alappākkam
5. Savarṇan Araiyan Madhurāntakan
6. Savarṇan Araiyan Chandraśēkharanāna Uttamacōḻa Aśalan
7. Savarṇan Pērāśiriyar Ādittadēvan Tiruvampalapperumān
8. Savarṇan Kāśyapa Kulōttuṅgacōḻa Maṅgalādhirāja
9. Savarṇan Tirumaṛaikkāvuḍaiyā

10 For a discussion of this, see M.R. Raghava Varier, *Jainism in Kerala*, a dissertation submitted to the Jawaharlal Nehru University, Delhi (unpublished), 1980. See also P.K. Gopalakrishnan, *Jainamatam Kēraḷattil* (Kottayam: Sahithya Pravarthaka Sahakaranasamgham, 2012).

11 For the facsimile and the relevant portion in the Anamalai inscription of Māṛan Cataiyan, see Devi, *Medicine in South India*, plate facing page 191.

There are references to *āturaśālais*, hospitals, attached to several temples situated in villages all over the region, thereby implying the spread of the system of Āyurveda. We hear about several centres, including those at Śrīraṅgam, Tanjāvūr, Tiruviśalūr, Tirumukkūṭal, Tiruntudēvankuṭi, Vēmbattūr, and so forth. The earliest one among these was at Devarayapettai in Pāpanāśam Taluk, Tanjavur.[12] The temple at Tirumukkūṭal has yielded a lengthy record dated in the sixth regnal year (1067 CE) of the Cōḻa king Vīrarājēndra, which furnishes much valuable data regarding the nature and content of the medical services provided by the institution (Figure 7.1).[13] The Vedic *śāla* (educational institute) had, in all, 3 teachers and 40 students. There were experts of the *Āgamas* and *tantras*, 10 *Mahāpañcarātras*, 3 *Śaiva Brāhmaṇas*, and 5 *Vaikhānasas*. The Vīracōḻan *āturaśālai* was meant exclusively for the teachers and students of the Vedic school attached to the temple. It was a fully equipped hospital as is clear from the document, under the physician Savarṇan Aśvatthāmā Bhattāraka of Ālappākkam. There were 15 beds, 1 physician, 1 surgeon, 2 servants, 2 nurses, 1 barber, and 1 waterman. All the abovementioned functionaries as well as the teachers and students were entitled to the medical facilities provided in the *Vīracōḻan āturaśālai* attached to the Venkatēśa Perumāḷ Temple at Tirumukkūṭal. The inscriptions refer to various functionaries rendering services to the hospital, such as *vaidyan* and *ambaṭṭan* or *nāviśan* (barber), and also the entitlements enjoyed by these functionaries, such as *vaidyappaṅku* or *vaidyabhāgam* (physician's share); *vaidyabhōgam* (that which can be enjoyed by physicians); *vaidyavirutti* (property set apart for physician's duty); *vaidyakkāṇi* (donation to physician); *śallyabhōgam*, *śallyavirutti*, or *śalliyakriyābhōgam* (property set apart for surgical programs); *viṣabhōgam viṣavirutti*, or *viṣaharabhōgam* (property set apart for treatment of poison).

The available data in the temple inscriptions clearly indicate that the medical treatment was looked after by the physicians, while the surgical operations were done by barbers who, evidently, came from the lower sections of society. They were known differently as *ambaṣṭha*,

[12] Archaeological Survey of India, *Annual Report of South-Indian Epigraphy*, New Delhi: Archaeological Survey of India, 1924, 16.

[13] K.V. Subrahmanya Aiyar, 'The Tirumukkutal Inscription of Virarajendra'; Archaeological Survey of India, *Epigraphia Indica (EI)* 21 (1931–32): 200–49.

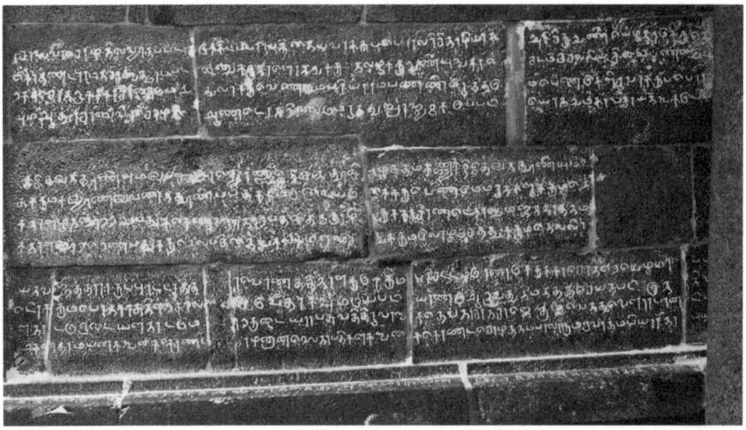

Figure 7.1 Thirumukkutal Inscription: Medicines Stored in the Hospital Attached to the Temple
Source: Author.

ampaṭṭa, *ampadyar*, *nāviśa*, and so forth. It is important to note in this connection, as we have already noted earlier, that surgical operations were carried out during the pre-modern times by barbers in the Western countries too.

As can be gleaned from the inscriptional records, physicians were settled in villages and they were endowed with landed property. For example, Śaravana Arayan Madhurāntakan was a great physician. He and his descendants enjoyed the rights of landed property for the medical service they rendered to the villages.[14] Kuntavai Pirāṭṭiyār purchased a certain land with a house for 12 *kasu* (coins) and gave the property to Śaravanan Arayan Candraśekharan for rendering medical service to the villagers. The Coḻa king Parāntaka gifted land as *brahmadeya* (property of Brahmins) to several Brahmins and this grant is recorded in an inscription from the twelfth century. The donees included astrologers, *paurāṇikas* (ancestors), physicians, and village servants, including barbers who attended to minor surgeries. In addition, a grant was given to a well-known physician named Ambulattādi Bhatta. One share of the land was given to the physician of the village Kumaramangala Vellathur during the 21st year of Pallava

[14] Archaeological Survey of India, *Annual Report of South Indian Epigraphy*, 16.

Nandivarman. Another Pallava record of the same period registers a grant of two shares for physicians. An inscription at Chidambaram of the thirteenth century lists the shares set apart for different institutions and communities in some newly formed villages. They included *vaidyar* (physician), *jātyambaṣṭa* (barber), surgeon, and midwives. A record dated 1264 CE registers a grant by King Sundara Pāṇḍyaṉ to some Brahmins and others. One-and-three-fourth share was given to a physician, half was for a ampadyar (barber, surgeon), three-fourth of the share for a *vīṇankolli*, and three-eighth of the share for a barber. Another gift of the thirteenth century CE included one share to *vaidyabhoga* (property set apart for a physician), entitled to Cēnan Koyil, who was a physician of high status in society. He is the donor of 100 sheep for a perpetual lamp in a temple. Arayan Uttamacōḻan was a barber and surgeon. He received a grant of one *veli* and four *mas* of land and a house at Vēmbattūr from the elder sister of Rājāraja Cōḻan for his surgical services (*śalyakriyābhoga*).[15] An inscription at Uttaramērūr in Chenkelpet district refers to the appointment of a physician for treating the cases of poisoning. The land donated to him was called *viṣaharabhoga* (property set aside for a physician of poisons). The same practices were continued by the Nāyaks and the Maraṭhas during their rule in Tamil Nadu. During the Maratha period, there were 5,783 villages in the Maratha principality of Tanjore and each village had a hereditary physician who enjoyed a share in the harvest of the village and one and a half acres of wet land.

From the available data, we are able to know certain facts about the nature and content of the Āyurvedic treatment during the medieval period in South India. First, the distribution pattern of the epigraphic documents indicates that the system had spread widely at the village level in the region. At the same time, it has to be remembered that we get information about the temple-centred Brahminical settlements only. No doubt, non-Brahminical settlements were in existence in the region but we are not sure whether the system was practised there too. Second, there were *āturaśālais*, hospitals, attached to the temples for providing medical services to the various groups. Thus, at certain places where there was a Vedic centre, the students and teachers were entitled to enjoy the services of the hospitals. Some other places had hospitals where the service was available for the villagers. Third, various personnel, including the *vaidya*, physicians,

[15] Vaili and mā are units of measurement.

surgeons, nurses, gatherers of herbal medicines, and other attendants who prepared the medicines, and so forth, were mostly Brahmins who looked after the medical treatment while the surgery was, as a rule, done by the barbers. These barbers were known differently as *ambaṣṭan, ampaṭṭan, nāviśan, prayōgattaraiyan*, and so forth. Fourth, there were arrangements for preparing and storing medicines at some centres. Some other centres purchased them according to the need of the hour from among the available places. Fifth, the *āturaśālais* was established by generous grants in the form of land and money by rich and powerful persons, often members of the ruling families or kings themselves. Service personnel were given entitlements in the form of landed property and money for the services rendered by them. The medicines prepared in the *āturaśālais* were named according to the classical texts of Āyurveda. Sixth, and more importantly, there were some centres of learning the science, such as the one at Thiruvaduthurai where the *Carakasamhita* and the *Aṣṭāṅgahṛdaya* were taught. These centres were responsible for the spread and perpetuation of the system of Āyurvedic medicine and practice in the region irrespective of the political changes that were taking place from time to time at the regional and local levels.

Medical Institutions

There were schools meant for medical education. An inscription of Vikram Chola (1121 CE) refers to a centre of learning in Thiruvaduthurai. Among the persons to be fed in the *maṭha* (residence of Brahmins) of that place were students of grammar and those who studied the *Carakasamhita* and Vāgbhaṭa's *Aṣṭāṅgahṛdaya*. A record of Parakesari Varman registers the sale of a land for the maintenance of a free dispensary. Another record of the same period mentions the sale of a house site to make up the deficit for an *āturaśālai* in Tanjavur.[16] Parakesari Varman granted remission of taxes for the maintenance of an *āturaśālai* on the northern bank of the river at Tiruppuṇaiyūr. Kunthavai Pirattiyar established a free dispensary in the memory of her father, Rājarāja Cōḻan.

[16] Varier, *History of Āyurveda*, 301–2. Table 7.1 lists the remuneration given to various staff members of a medical institution.

Table 7.1 Remuneration Given to Staff Members of the Medical Institution

Remuneration of staff	Paddy	Money
1. Physician	90 Kalam[17] paddy	8 Ponkasu
2. Surgeon	30 Kalam paddy	2 Ponkasu
3. Servants	30 Kalam	2 Ponkasu
4. Nurses	30 Kalam	½ Ponkasu
5. Barber	15 Kalam	Nil
6. Water Man	15 Kalam	Nil

Source: Varier, *History of Āyurveda*, 301–2.

Medicines were prepared, stored, and distributed in some villages for the village folk. Epigraphic records give us the names of such medicines prepared in the villages. Some of such medicines were:

1. Brahma Rasāyana
2. Gomūtraharītaki
3. Grandare
4. Balākeraṇḍatailam
5. Pañcakatailam
6. Laśunairaṇḍāditailam
7. Uttamakarṇāditailam
8. Vilwādi Ghṛtam
9. Maṇḍūkara Vaṭika
10. Travatti
11. Vimala
12. Sunethri
13. Tāmrādi
14. Vajrakalpa
15. Kalpaka Lavaṅga
16. Pūrakakhaṇḍam

The above list gives us valuable information about the nature of medicines and the treatment prevalent in the Tamil south in the period under consideration. First, the medicines were prepared strictly following the method and ingredients of the classical texts. Second, the mode of treatment was hospital-oriented and not domestic as interpreted by some scholars. Third, preparations with metals such as *tāmra* (copper) also were in common use in addition to the herbal

[17] Kalam is an old measurement used for grains.

plants. Fourth, and more importantly, all categories of medicines, including *rasāyana*, *ghṛta* (ghee), *vaṭika* (pills), *taila* (oil), and so forth, were made available for the patients.

As gleaned from the epigraphic records, this tradition was continued in the subsequent period too by the Kākatiyas, the Yādavas, the Vijayanagaras, and the Nāyaks. The Chebrolu inscription of Jaya dated Śaka year 1135 (1213 CE), the chief of the elephant troop of the Kākatiya king Gaṇapati mentions a vaidya as a recipient of a grant of land.[18] Similarly, the Thana plates of the time of the Yadava King Ramachandra dated Śaka year 1194 (1272 CE) informs that Hemādri, superintendant of the elephant troops and the chief minister of the king, was a scholar and a physician. Hemādri is well known as the author of two commentaries—the *Āyurvedarasāyana* of the *Aṣṭāṅgahṛdaya* and the *Kaivalyadīpaka* of *Muktāphala*—and an encyclopaedic work, the *Caturvarga Cintāmaṇi*.[19] A stone pillar inscription from Malkapuram in Andhra Pradesh informs us that Viśvēśvarācārya provided a grant for the establishment of a centre of education attached to the *maṭha*.[20] The centre included a *prasūtiśāla* (maternity house), an *ārōgyaśāla* (hospital), and a *viprasatra* (inn). An arrangement was also made to provide the services of a physician at the institution.[21] Plates at the Government Museum, Chennai, dated Śaka year 1346 (1424 CE) of Śrīgiribhūpāla of the Vijayanagara dynasty mention the name of a great scholar and physician, Govinda Paṇḍita, 'who had seen the further shore of the Ocean of Ayurveda and the *vedāṅgas*'.[22] The Somālipuram Grant of Virūpākṣa dated Śaka year 1389 (1467 CE) mentions the name of Virūpākṣārya, a great physician and scholar in connection with a land grant.[23] The Padmaneri Grant

[18] E. Hultzsch, 'Chebrolu Inscription of Jaya, Śaka samvat, 1135'; Archaeological Survey of India, *EI*, 5 (1898–9): 150.

[19] Barnett D Lionell, 'Thana Plates of the Time of the Yadava king Ramachandra, śaka 1194'; Archaeological Survey of India, *EI*, 13 (1915–16): 198–206, lines 39–41.

[20] B. Rama Rao, 'Contribution of Andhra to Ayurveda in Sanskrit', *Bulletin of International Institute of Hindu Medicine*, 1978, 3 (1–4): 8.

[21] Zysk, *Asceticism and Healing* in Ancient India, 45.

[22] M. Narayanaswami Ayyar, 'Madras Museum plates of Śrīgiribhūpāla'; Archaeological Survey of India, *EI*, 8 (1905–6), 306–17.

[23] K.V. Subrahmania Iyer, 'Somalipuram Grant of Virūpākṣa'; Archaeological Survey of India, *EI*, 17 (1923–4), 193–204.

of Venkata I dated Śaka year 1520 (1598 CE) also makes a similar statement about a land grant to a physician named Paramasvāmi Vaidyan.[24] The Nagardhan Plates of Swamirāja mention the name of Sāmasvāmi, a *hastivaidya*, physician of elephants.[25] The Pithapuram plates of Vīracōḍa mention vaidya, physician, *ambaṣṭa*, surgeon, and *viṣavādi*, a specialist in toxicology, among those who received land grant from the authorities.[26] During the beginning of the seventeenth century, Raghunātha Nayak (1616 CE) donated 6 *paṇam* (coins) along with 150 *kuḻi*[27] of land for Mārgasahāya Paṇḍitar, a famous physician.

Developments in Medieval Kerala

The Velan medicine-men as functionaries in the village community of Kerala were practising physicians with a knowledge of indigenous medicine. Their womenfolk as rural midwives used some instruments and small blades in their profession. However, they did not follow the tradition of *śalyatantra* (surgery as a technical subject) as described in the classical texts. An indigenous, non-classical, and hereditary tradition of midwifery was their source of knowledge. Later, due to the increase of population and a corresponding growth in the number of village settlements, the services of the community of Velans could not be distributed equally to cater to the needs of all the villages. In places where the Velans were absent, other communities took to their healing techniques. Thus, in the erstwhile Taluk of Kuṟumbranāḍ there were the Paravas and their womenfolk, *paratti*, who rendered medical services to the village community. Similarly, Vaṇṇāns were practitioners of medicine in the erstwhile Taluk of Eranad. In Palghat Taluk, the hereditary professions of Maṇṇāns included medicine in addition to dancing, singing, washing, and treatment of cattle. All these communities followed the scientific

[24] V. Natesa Aiyer, 'Padmaneri Grant of Venkata I'; Archaeological Survey of India, *EI*, 16 (1921–2), 289.

[25] V.V. Mirashi, 'Nagardhan Plates of Svamiraja'; Archaeological Survey of India, *EI*, 28 (1949–50), 1–11.

[26] H. Krishna Sastri, 'Pithapuram Plates of Venkata I'; Archaeological Survey of India, *EI*, 5 (1898–9), 70.

[27] Kuḷi is a measurement of land.

system of Āyurveda, thereby implying a total acculturation or Sanskritization of the local tradition of healing. At the same time, they did not give up their hereditary local traditions of the art of healing. A notable difference between the Velan and the Parava groups was that while the Velans were full-time medicine-men with their magico-religious rites, the Paravas took up other professions, such as fishing, shell processing, masonry, and so forth. Interestingly, both the communities and their womenfolk shared the same non-classical local knowledge of medicine and the indigenous and rural labour practices. The system with its local traditions of medical services continued to survive for several centuries in the rural villages of Kerala until it was totally marginalized and replaced by the modern hospital system by about the last quarter of the twentieth century without leaving any trace behind.

A notable feature of the curative practices of the communities of Velan, Paravan, and Maṇṇān at a later stage was the influence of the classical knowledge of the traditions of Vāgbhaṭa and the Aṣṭavaidyans. It is equally important to note that this was not a one-way traffic of cultural influence. The Aṣṭavaidyans of Kerala, who strictly followed the tradition of Vāgbhaṭa, were not free from the influences of indigenous local traditions. Each hereditary family of Aṣṭavaidyans was keen in composing therapeutic texts on various aspects of Āyurvedic treatment. These texts are replete with portions that are not found in the classics but are familiar to the local tradition. In some contexts, as in the case of *Ālattūr Maṇipravāḷam*, the pharmacopoeia of one of the oldest Aṣṭavaidya families, it is stated that 'this is an advice', thereby indicating that the portion is from some local tradition, probably from that of the village medicine.[28] Apart from these, there are several portions in these texts that dilate upon the indigenous and traditional modes of treatment peculiar to Kerala, such as *Dhāra*, *Navarakkiḻi*, *Piḻiccil*, and so forth. It can be maintained on the basis of these practices that the local and non-classical traditions of Kerala have contributed substantially to the rich and varied heritage of the science of Āyurveda.[29]

Medicinal practices and healing techniques are developed in human societies strictly in order to cater to some physical needs.

[28] M.R. Raghava Varier et al., *Ālattūr Maṇipravāḷam*, text with commentary (Kottakkal: Arya Vaidya Sala, 2009).

[29] For a learned observation on this aspect of Kerala tradition, see P.K. Warrier, *Pādamudrakaḷ* (Mal.) (Kottakkal: Arya Vaidya Sala, 2002), 114–16.

Medieval society in Kerala with its peculiar form of political set-up of the territorial Swarūpam ruling families and their retinue required some techniques of healing. These territorial rulers with their limited resources could not abstain from encroaching the neighbouring territories for more and more resources. At the same time, they could not and did not maintain a standing army. Local chiefs, appointed by the ruling Swarūpams in their respective areas with specific duties and entitlements, were responsible for supplying the stipulated number of fighters at the time of military operations. Military operations had to be carried out with fighters who were at the beck and call of the local chiefs. This political system called for some arrangements in the local village settlements for the development of training centres for martial groups and this resulted in the formation of the Kaḷari system and its particular knowledge of *marma vidya*, the knowledge of cardinal points in the human body. These Kaḷaris were the institutional base of a highly developed form of training in gymnastics and martial techniques with a well-organized curriculum and syllabi. The traditional teachers with the knowledge and expertise in the *marma vidya* lore treated serious and dangerous fracture of bones and impairments of the cardinal points. It has to be noted in this connection that this local lore is different in many respects from the *marma* concept of the classical tradition of Āyurveda.[30] Further, differences are many between one local tradition and the others. Interestingly enough, there are numerous texts pertaining to this branch of traditional knowledge in all our manuscript libraries and some of them are available in print both in Tamil as well as in Malayalam.[31] These texts deal in great detail with the treatment of the fracture of bones and the impairment of limbs. This branch of knowledge is a valuable contribution of a non-classical tradition of Kerala. Regular beneficiaries of this system of healthcare in the traditional society of Kerala were members of the local militia and the communities that were engaged in climbing of coconut trees, palm trees, and so forth. It is worth noting that this traditional knowledge was formulated and codified by communities other than Nambudiris or the Aṣṭavaidyans.

[30] The classical texts in Āyurveda refer to the *marma*, cardinal points in the human body but leave it at that stage without giving details.

[31] See, for example, M. Kunjukrishnan Nadar, *Marmasasthrapeethika* (Thiruvanantapuram: Mangalodyam Book Depot, 1975).

Another area enriched by non-classical traditional knowledge is the treatment for cases of poisons. Kerala is considered in myths and legendary accounts as a place infested with poisonous reptiles. It is not at all surprising that a systematic knowledge of poisons and an efficient mode of treatment for snake bite and other accidents was produced and practised in Kerala. A considerable amount of knowledge has been recorded, thanks to the laborious task undertaken by private households.[32] Traditional *gurukulas*, such as the Kodungallur palace, were keen on including *viṣavaidyam*, toxicology treatment for poison, in their traditional curriculum for higher studies.[33] It is also important that specialization in branches, such as *netracikitsa*, ophthalmology, and *bālacikitsa*, treatment for children, and so forth, attained high status during the pre-colonial epoch of history.

During the long period of several centuries of unbroken tradition of these rural settlements, some areas, such as the forest-clad hill tracts of Wayanad and Idukki-Munnar high ranges, were cut off from the rest of the regions due to reasons including the hostile nature of the terrain, epidemics, and so on. The aboriginal groups of these hill tracts were confined to their locality with the least amount of relation with the world outside. These groups developed a separate tradition of tribal medicine, consisting mainly of wild herbs that are available only in the ecosystem of their respective regions. Thus, the Kuṛicciyas, Kuṛumas, and Paṇiyas of Wayanad, and the Maṉṉāns and Mutuvas of the high ranges have some knowledge of herbs and their curative properties. Practices of these tribal medicines were, until recently, confined to their own limited circles with the age-old tradition of preparation.

A common feature shared by all these non-classical and local traditions is that they are all meant for individuals suffering from various ailments. Therefore, the treatment was domestic in nature in the spheres of preparation and consumption of medicines. Large scale production in factories and an organized and market-oriented network of distribution was not their interest at the level of conception; nor was it necessary or possible in the existing social formation.

[32] M.P. Purushothaman Nair, *Thaliyola Granthasuchi* (Catalogue of Palm leaf manuscripts; Mal.), 2 Vols (Kerala: Calicut University, 1985).

[33] Koyippalli Parameswara Kurup, *Suvarnayugam* (Calicut: K. R. Brothers, 1957). The book narrates the reminiscences of a writer about the Kodungallur palace, a high place of learning in the pre-colonial period.

The contemporary market with its potential omnipresence has entered into the sphere and brought about a shift in the management of ailment using medicines of non-classical traditions and tribal lore. Voluntary organizations and NGOs are also active as clients for the fruits of this service. The present scenario of medical treatment is characterized by the dominating presence of an alliance of three forces—medicine, market, and media. This alliance has brought about a phase of transition. An important result seems to be that two factors of medical treatment have been conveniently set apart or nullified—the physician and the patient. However, it is not yet time to evaluate the merits and demerits of this change.

The classical and the non-classical are conventionally understood as belonging to distinctive realms of cultural tradition. According to this view, the classical is supra-local, pervasive, and dominant, whereas the non-classical is local, passive, and amenable. What is more important is the mode of storage and retrieval, particularly in the case of a scientific knowledge. The classical tradition in most of the cases is recorded and transmitted by means of written texts, while the non-classical is thought to have been preserved in memory and transmitted orally. This, however, need not be taken as a rigid rule, for there are instances of classical tradition, such as the Vedic lore preserved in memory and transmitted orally. Non-classical traditions such as the local knowledge of *marma vidya*, as distinct from the classical concept of *marma*s in the human body, is recorded and transmitted in the form of written texts. Differences apart, the two realms share in common certain features that are decisive in shaping the contours of their form and content. Both the spheres are developed as the results of long processes of meticulous data collection, constant observation, careful examination, and scrupulous verification. They are functioning not in watertight compartments but in open social spaces and, therefore, both the traditions tend to engage in interactions with each other. These interfaces render them with opportunities for reconciliation with other traditions and world views. Encounters of classical Āyurveda with regional traditions have resulted in mutual borrowing of techniques and strategies and, therefore, it may be a futile exercise to search for a pure form of the classical or the non-classical tradition. However, a search about the distinctiveness of these traditions is not out of place in the context of an enquiry into the transitional phases and shifts of paradigms of scientific traditions.

8

Experiment with Modernity

The Decline and Reawakening of Āyurveda

The Indian system of medicine was effective and suited to the local needs as in other areas of tradition. The British Raj, with its project of 'ordering difference' between India and the West, ruthlessly condemned it, describing the Indian traditional medicine as 'unscientific' and 'superstitious'.[1] G. Mukhopadhyaya has shown how Indian medical traditions were completely ignored and how Indian universities refused to provide a place for Āyurveda in their medical curriculum.[2] Still, a section of the European authorities, such as W. Adam, argued for 'a synthesis of exotic principles and local practices, European

[1] For a detailed discussion on the 'ordering of difference, see Thomas R. Metcalf, *Ideologies of the Raj* (Delhi: Cambridge University Press, 1998), 113–16.

[2] G. Mukhopadhyay, *History of Indian Medicine*, I (Calcutta University Press: Calcutta, 1923), 94.

theory and Indian experience'.[3] In *Report on Vernacular Education*, Adam opined that this could revive, invigorate, enlighten, and liberalize the native medical profession in the mofussil.[4]

A medical school was started in 1822 with the purpose of teaching both the Western and Indian systems of medicine. Medical classes were also started at the Calcutta Sanskrit School and the Calcutta Madrasa. Similar attempts were made in Bombay and Madras but they failed and died out before long due to the attitude of the authorities.

The setback to Āyurveda with the British occupation is generally explained as a result of the British policy towards the indigenous systems of knowledge and wisdom, including that of healthcare. Reasons from within, such as the craze regarding the newly appeared foreign elements and a neglect for indigenous things, have not been considered seriously. Further, the preparation of Āyurvedic medicines was a cumbersome process, whereas Western medicines, if at hand, were readily available from the hospitals and health centres. This saved clients from the difficult process of preparation of native medicine. Above all, the gurukula methods of teaching and learning of Āyurveda was a system that involved tremendous hardship for the students. The situation was aggravated with a hostile attitude of the British Raj towards native medicine.

However, an age-old tradition with a strong scientific base and a time-tested system of healing and healthcare could not simply die out even under the strongest of adverse attitudes. This is how a set of great masterminds appeared on the scene and upheld the cause of Āyurveda against all adverse forces. The activities of these masterminds started towards the end of the nineteenth century CE. Calcutta, which was the capital of the Indian colonial rule in the beginning, was a great centre of renaissance. Celebrated scholars and physicians, such as Gangadhara Ray (1799–1855), Yogendranath Sen (1871–1918), Ganganatha Sen (1877–1956), Haranachandra Chakraborthy (–1930), and Yaminibhushan Ray (1879–1925), were engaged in various activities for promoting the cause of Āyurveda. Gangadhara Ray trained a band of efficient disciples and published a commentary for the *Carakasamhita* with a view to emphasizing the philosophical aspect

[3] W. Adam quoted in Deepak Kumar, *Science and the Raj 1857–1905*. (Delhi: Oxford India Paper Backs 1997), 52.

[4] W. Adam, *Report on Vernacular Education* (Calcutta, 1868), 322–3.

and practical efficacy of the great work. Yogendranath Sen, a disciple of Gangadhara Ray, also prepared a commentary for *Carakasamhita*. Ganganatha Sen was a scholar-physician who made it a point to explain the principles of Āyurveda according to the principles of modern medicine. At the same time, he adhered to the genuine spirit of the indigenous science of health. He learnt modern medicine from the Calcutta Medical College and in 1929 he was invited by Madanmohan Malavya to be appointed as the dean of the Faculty of Āyurveda at the Benaras Hindu University (BHU). In 1932, he started the Āyurveda Mahavidyalaya in Calcutta in memory of his father. He was keen on updating the principles of Āyurveda. The *Pratyakṣaśārīra*, a textbook on anatomy incorporating modern and ancient understanding of the subject, is a great contribution of Gananath Sen. Similarly, he brought out a work on pathology entitled *Siddhāntanidānam*.

Haranachandra Chakraborthy concentrated mainly on surgery, following the methods of the *Suśrutasamhita*. He was famous in ophthalmic surgery. His commentary on the *Suśrutasamhita* entitled the *Suśrutartha Sandeepani* is much acclaimed for its scientific value.

Yaminibhushan Ray, a native of East Bengal, was a great Sanskrit scholar and a great physician. He was a product of the Calcutta Medical College. He chose to practise Āyurveda after getting trained under Kaviraj Mahopadhyaya Vijayaratna Sen. He established the Ashtanga Āyurveda College at Calcutta in 1916, and became the founder principal of that institution. His works include the *Rogavinishchaya*, the *Śālākyatantra*, the *Kaumāratantra*, and the *Viṣa Vijñāna*.

Sankardaji Pade (1866–1909) was born in Bombay as the son of a renowned astrologer, learned traditional Sanskrit, and then Āyurveda from Bhanu Vaidya Kulkarni. He published a journal called the *Rajavaidya*, which was changed afterwards to the *Aryabhiṣak*. Another Hindi journal, the *Sadvaidyakaustubham*, was also started by Pade. He wrote books on Vāgbhaṭa, Caraka, and so forth and on subjects such as *Bṛhannighaṇṭu* (dictionary), *Vanouṣadhiguṇādarśa* (account of forest herbs used in medicine), and so forth.

P.S. Varier (1869–1943) was born in south Malabar, Kerala, and received formal education in the traditional style and subjects such as Sanskrit grammar, poetry, and so forth. Then he joined the Kuttancheri Apphan Moosad, a member of an Aṣṭavaidya family, and studied Āyurveda in the gurukula model with all the hardships of that system. After completing the studies successfully, he practised Āyurveda at Kottakkal, where his family was settled. Soon, he became fully aware of the degenerated condition of the native medicines and their use. In 1902, Varier started a small establishment under the name Aryavaidyasala for preparing and distributing genuine Āyurvedic medicines to needy people. It is this humble institution that has now grown to the status of the headquarters of the science of Āyurveda. Varier came in contact with Dr Varghese of Manjeri and acquired working knowledge of modern medicine from him. In 1903, he took the leadership role in establishing the Aryavaidya Samajam, which spearheaded various programmes for the development of Āyurveda. The Samajam served as a common platform for Āyurvedic physicians to unite and to act for updating and propagating the science of Āyurveda. Simultaneously, he started a journal, the *Dhanvantari*, in 1903, which was an open forum for scientific discussions and exchange of ideas. In 1917, Varier started the Aryavaidya Pāṭhaśāla at Calicut and it was later shifted to Kottakkal. He started a charitable hospital at Kottakkal, which provided the much-needed service of Āyurvedic and modern treatment for the public. Considering the value of the great contributions of the scholar-physician, the Government of India conferred upon him the title of Vaidyaratnam in the year 1933. He wrote books such as the *Bṛhadchārīra* and the *Aṣṭāngaśārīra*, and numerous articles on various issues. A poet, playwright, and composer, Varier authored several dramas to be staged by the ParamaŚiva-Vilāsam Nāṭyasaṅgham, which was established by him in 1913.

Swami Laxmiram (1873–1939) of Rajasthan studied Āyurveda from the Jaipur Āyurveda College and joined Dwarakanath Sen in Calcutta for higher training. He was soon established as a professor of Āyurveda and later started a clinic and also an endowment trust for the publication of books on Āyurveda.

Yadavji Trikramji Acharya (1887–1956), born at Porbandar in Gujarat, learned Sanskrit and Āyurveda from his father who was the court physician of the *rajasaheb* of Porbandar. He also learned Unani and became the first principal of the Āyurveda College at BHU. Joining P.M. Mehta, he worked substantially to start the Gujarat Āyurveda University. The *Madhukośa* commentary of *Madhavanidana*, the *Āyurveda Deepika* commentary of the *Carakasamhita*, the *Nibandha* commentary of the *Suśrutasamhita*, and several other volumes were produced by Yadavji.

P.M. Mehta (1889–1979), born in Gujarat, studied modern medicine and Āyurveda. He was a professor of surgery at BHU and became famous as an Āyurvedic surgeon. He has written a commentary for the *Suśrutasamhita*. There are also significant contributions to his credit, such as the *aupasaṅgika rogas*, *jīvanu vijñāna*, mutra roga, swasthya *Vijñāna*, and *vaidyakiya subhaṣita sahitya*.

Damodar Sharma Gaud (1909–1984) was an eminent faculty member of BHU. He wrote several works on Āyurveda, such as the *Āyurveda Darshanasangraha*, *Surgical Ethics in Āyurveda*, and so forth. Similarly, P.V. Sharma (b. 1920), a most eminent Āyurvedic scholar of the twentieth century, is a product of BHU. He served the Bihar government as the deputy director of Indian medicine. He established the PG Institute in BHU. He was appointed professor of Dravyaguna. He has served the Bihar government in several official positions. His substantial contribution to the science of Āyurveda include English translations of the *Carakasamhita* (in five volumes) and the *Suśrutasamhita* (in four volumes).

A pattern is discernible in the programmes and projects of the above-mentioned renaissance personalities who walked in the forefront of the resurrection of the indigenous science of Āyurveda. One of the common features is their acquaintance with and proficiency in modern medicine. Almost all of them either studied modern medicine formally or got training from competent medical practitioners. A second feature is their proficiency in the textual knowledge of Āyurveda and the resultant competence in commenting on classical texts. A third quality of these pioneers is their keenness in propagating the science of Āyurveda to the new generations. All of the above-mentioned scholar-physicians engaged themselves in teaching Āyurveda with the result that they had a large number of disciples; a few of them started clinics and produced and distributed medicine according to the textual prescriptions. The meaning and significance of these activities from various corners and viewpoints would not be clear unless and until they are placed in their historical background. The time of the activities of these scholar-physicians was vibrant with the fervour of the Indian national movement, the waves of which had reached every nook and corner of the subcontinent. People from all walks of life were encouraged and inspired by the call for a national awakening. It was against this historical context that the zealous attempts of the masters of Āyurveda were staged. All of the great personalities mentioned above were great scholars and expert physicians who contributed richly to one or two or more fields of activities, such as writing books, engaging new methods in teaching, modernizing the methods of preparation of medicines, modalities of treatment, and so on.

Interestingly enough, Vaidyaratnam P.S. Varier contributed richly to all the areas of the activities mentioned earlier. First, he started an establishment to supply genuine medicines for the needy. This was an effective step towards remedying the inherent weakness of the native medicine in the period under consideration. Second, he started a journal, the *Dhanwantari*, for propagating the ideas and ideals of Āyurveda and to provide a platform for discussing issues and problems of healthcare in general. Third, he was successful in starting a centre for teaching Āyurveda with a view to minimizing the difficulties of students who chose to study the subject and also to modernize the subject of study according to an updated curriculum and syllabi. Fourth, he was successful in unifying the practitioners of Āyurveda in Kerala under the banner of Āyurveda Samajam and also providing a common platform for the physicians to discuss in detail the problems and issues confronted by the subject. Varier did this when the idea of a united Kerala was not even envisaged by politicians and social workers. Further, he established a manufacturing centre and supplied genuine medicine for the needy, since he was aware of the need of the hour.

Concluding Observations

The origin and development of the indigenous science of healing and healthcare in India is often traced back to the Harappan culture of the third–second millennium BCE. An acute scarcity of reliable data prevents us from making meaningful statements about the nature and method of healing and healthcare in that distant past, except some objects, such as asphalt with medicinal properties or one or two skulls, suggesting the marks of trepanation. The Rgvedic hymns are the earliest sources now available, which contain useful information regarding any considerable fund of knowledge of diseases and their treatment. Vedic medicine is often described as 'magico-religious', thereby implying that the art of healing and healthcare as referred to in the Vedic hymns involved both the use of medicine as well as the ritualistic chanting of hymns. The early phase is characterized by primitive methods of nature treatment, that is, curing ailments by natural materials, such as water, heat, fire, and earth. The *Aithareya Brāhmaṇa* (1, 5: 2) states that fire or heat is the medicine to restore life. The same text makes a noteworthy observation that rainwater charged with the sun's rays is medicine or a potent drink. The *Śatapatha Brāhmaṇa* (5, 1: 46) states that 'within water is medicine'. The Vedic seers had clear knowledge of toxicology and they knew that the remedy was sour things, such as tamarind, curd, and so forth. The *Aithareya Brāhmaṇa* (2, 8: 4) reports a case of Mithra and Varuna, who neutralized intoxication by curd. This need not mean that herbal medicines were not known to the Vedic seers. There are some portions that regarded soma as the king of creepers and medicinal plants. *Śatapatha Brāhmaṇa* (3, 1: 1–7) refers to ointments prepared out of plants and trees for sores and itches.

From the foregoing account, it is possible to delineate certain characteristic features of the knowledge of Vedic medicine and the art of healing. First, healthcare during the Vedic period extending to a long span of time can be understood as belonging to two distinctive stages. The early stage was characterized by the practice of natural healing, that is, treatment by natural elements, such as water. *Bhiṣaks*, a section in the society with some amount of specialization, were the practitioners. Their art of healing included medicine supplemented by magical rites and incantations of hymns. Second, specialization in the Vedic medical lore presupposes some amount of systematic organization of the knowledge of the science of medicine accumulated during the long period from 1000 BCE to the middle of the first millennium BCE. Third, the medicinal knowledge of the *bhiṣaks* was supported and supplemented by the auxiliary knowledge of the human anatomy, probably accumulated from the experience in the sacrificial rituals. Fourth, there was a steady growth of knowledge of plant and plant life, including a vast amount of medicinal lore pertaining to the herbal plants. Fifth, and most significantly, there was a parallel development of a tradition of rational thinking of the Nyāya, the Vaiśeṣika, and the Sānkhya schools of philosophy. Rational explanations of diseases and their healing can be understood as a result of this tradition. This was further supported by the heterodox philosophical thinking, which was free from the hold of fear of Vedic deities and demons. This element of reason and rational thinking was instrumental in bringing about radical change, and a shift of paradigm in the indigenous knowledge of the science of Āyurveda.

Significantly enough, Vedic healing involved both the medicinal treatment and a preliminary form of surgery. For example, a reed was used as catheter in the treatment of the retention of urine. Cauterization with caustic medicines was in vogue. Sand was in use in order to stop the flow of blood from the uterus or from a wound. It is known from the hymns that some kind of resin was applied to wounds for preventing them from bleeding and also to aid in the process of healing. Ointments and dyes were applied to the skin and a certain plant was in use for promoting the growth of hair. Water was a medicine used for the treatment of several diseases, both internal and external.

The topic of the nature and content of the Vedic perfomance of magico-religious healing has received careful attention from scholars and it has been shown what exactly the term meant in the context of medicine. Close reading and proper understanding of the meaning of hymns in the *Rgveda* prove that plants and herbs were put under rigorous scrutiny and their important features and qualities noted. The technique was a method in the form of recording valuable facts and this is an example of the very beginning of the empirical mode of the practice of medicine. This can be taken as an example as suggested by a recent authority as 'the very beginning of the Indian's empirical mode of thought'.[1] According to the clear information culled out from our sources, it is evident that there existed some kind of classificatory system of thinking. The technique of diagnosis and prognosis illustrate the importance given to the recording of observable facts.

Heterodox sections, such as the Jaina and the Buddhist ones, brought in new approaches and methods in the traditional art of healing and healthcare. Buddha, the Enlightened One, explained that the cause of mankind's suffering was eight-fold: bile (*pitta*), phlegm (*sehma*), wind (*vāta*), and their combination (*sannipāta*) are the primary causes. In addition to these, there are (*a*) changes of the seasons, (*b*) stress of unusual activities, (*c*) going out hastily at night and being bitten by a snake, and (*d*) the results of action. It is worth noting that this eight-fold formula of causation of diseases includes the three peccant humours. The relation between these and the theory of *tridoṣa*, central to Āyurveda, is unmistakable.

The gradual development of the Buddhist monastic tradition of medicine resulted in the codification of medical knowledge, and the rules pertaining to the use of drugs and treatments for specific ailments. Such rules were present in a large part in the early Āyurvedic medical treatises. The congruence of these approaches strongly suggests a common origin for both the Buddhist monastery and the early Āyurvedic tradition. Legendary accounts and the Pāli texts clearly show that the Buddhist monasteries played a significant role in the development of medical ethics. In addition to these, the Buddhist monasteries provided an institutional base for the medical treatment of the *bhikṣus* as per the advice and leadership of the Buddha, the Enlightened One himself.

Systematic recordering and scientific codifying of the rich fund of knowledge that accumulated in the course of a very long period was perhaps the invaluable contribution of the Samhitas. Further, these

[1] Zysk, *Medicine in the Veda*, 9.

texts were instrumental in fixing the nature and modalities of various forms of treatments for different kinds of diseases. It is in the Samhitas that we come across for the first time a certain amount of specialization in medicine as well as surgery, including rhinoplasty. The *Suśrutasamhita* in general and the section on *Śālākyatantra* in particular acquire added relevance and importance against the historical facts about the ancient Indian tradition of jurisprudence at least from the time of the Mauryan rule. The *Dharmaśastra* texts, such as the *Manusmṛti*, mention the 10 places of the human body where punishment for offences were to be given to non-Brahmins, which included the nose in addition to the eyes, ears, hands, tongue, and so forth. Coming to the later periods, during the Mughal and the sultanate periods, the mutilation of the nose continued as a form of punishment. It is clear from the charts prepared by surgeons of the nineteenth century that women were the patients in a large number of cases. The amputation of the nose was a social malaise in India, which was used as means of settling personal grudges, and as a punitive measure for misdeeds, misbehaviour, as well as the violation of marital sanctity. According to some charts prepared by the practitioners of rhinoplasty in South India, in the nineteenth century 63 patients out of 100 cases were women.[2] Thus, it may not be improbable to assume that the techniques, including the rhinoplastic surgical treatments, were conceived and developed in order to cater to some contemporary social needs. References to cataract surgery are many in the early Buddhist texts, which were translated into Chinese from the original Buddhist canonical texts. If we go by the dates mentioned by the scholar for the transmission of knowledge of cataract surgery to China, it seems to suggest in unequivocal terms that cataract surgery was known to the surgeons prior to the composition of the *Uttaratantra* or that the dates of composition of the text had to be pushed back in time prior to the date of the composition of that text, that is, earlier than the fourth century CE.[3] It may be added in this connection that the Samhitas of *ācaryās*, such as Kāśyapa, Bheḷa, and Hārīta, brought in the idea of specialization in the knowledge and practice of treatment for diseases, including mental disorders (*kaumārabhṛtya* for children's ailments), and so on.

[2] Majumdar and Mukherjee, *Essays on History of Medicine*, 67–87.

[3] Majumdar and Mukherjee, *Essays on History of Medicine*.

The Mauryan period witnessed an unprecedented spread of the indigenous system of treatment in the whole of the subcontinent and also in the neighbouring areas, thanks to the efforts of the emperor Ashoka. This resulted in the encounter of the system of Āyurveda that gradually developed in the Ganga–Yamuna doab and the local and regional knowledges of healing in different parts of the subcontinent. The result was, in all probability, the mutual influence of both the systems. The system introduced by Ashoka was, in all probability, the one developed into a science in the Buddhist *vihāras* of the northern territories. Ashoka's interest in the Buddhist *saṅghas* and their programmes is too well known to call for any further explanation. It has been suggested on the basis of the Pāli and Sanskrit sources that the shift of paradigm in the ancient Indian healing and healthcare into an 'empirico-rational medicine' was an achievement of the ascetics in the Buddhist *vihāras*.[4] One or two points in this regard appear to be noteworthy in this cultural transaction. First, the local Tamil tradition came under the influence of a Prakrit tradition of heterodox groups. As a rule, the earliest phase of the science of Āyurveda is traced to the Vedic hymns, mainly the *Atharvaveda* and much less from the *Rgveda*, which contain numerous references to a medicinal lore mixed with myth, magic, and miracle. Here, in the Mauryan sources, the reference is to an instituted process of *cikitsa* (treatment).

Epigraphic documents pertaining to the relevant period provide us with certain facts about the nature and content of the Āyurvedic treatment during the medieval period in all the regions, including South India upto Sri Lanka. First, the documents indicate that the system had spread widely at a village level in all the regions. Second, there were *āturaśālais*, hospitals attached to the temples for providing medical services to the various groups. At certain places, where there were vedic centres, the students and teachers were entitled to enjoy the services of the hospitals, while at other places the medical service was available for the entire village community. Third, physicians, surgeons, nurses, as well as gatherers of herbal medicines and other attendants, who prepared the medicine and so on, were appointed, and these service sections were entitled to receive income according to the nature of their job. Physicians looked after the medicinal treatment, while the surgery was, as a rule, done by the barbers.

4 Zysk, *Asceticism and Healing in Ancient India*, 21–2.

Fourth, at some centres there were arrangements for preparing and storing medicines. Some other centres purchased them according to the need of the hour. Fifth, the *āturaśālai*s were established by generous grants in the form of land as well as money by rich and powerful persons, often members of the royal families or kings themselves. Service personnel were given entitlements in the form of landed property and money for the services rendered by them. Finally, and more importantly, there were centres of learning the science of Āyurveda and these centres were responsible for the spread and perpetuation of the system of Āyurvedic medicine and its practice in the region irrespective of the political changes that were taking place from time to time.

The setback of Āyurveda during the colonial rule has to be explained not only by the hostile attitude of the British Raj towards the native medical practice but also by reasons from within, such as the craze towards the newly emerging foreign elements and a neglect for indigenous things, which has not yet been considered seriously. However, an age-old tradition with a strong scientific base and a time-tested system of healing and healthcare could not simply die out even under the strongest of adverse attitudes. A set of great masterminds appeared on the scene and upheld the cause of Āyurveda above all adverse forces. The activities of these masterminds started towards the end of the nineteenth century CE.

It is interesting to note that elements of the pattern are discernible in the programmes and projects of the above-mentioned renaissance personalities, who walked in front of the resurrection of the indigenous science. One such common features is the proficiency of the nationalist experts of modern medicine. Almost all of them had either studied modern medicine formally or got training from competent medical practitioners. A second feature is their knowledge of the classical texts of Āyurveda and their resultant competence in commenting on them. A third quality of these pioneering stalwarts is their keenness in propagating the science of Āyurveda among the new generations. All of the above-mentioned scholar–physicians engaged themselves in teaching Āyurveda with the result that they had a large number of disciples. A few of them started clinics, and produced and distributed medicines according to the textual prescriptions. The activities mentioned above brought in a series of changes in the areas related to the knowledge of Āyurveda. The most popular among these were the changes from kitchen preparation to bottled medicines and from traditional healing at home to the hospital system of treatment. In the field of medical education, the age-old gurukula system was replaced by the newly emerging college system with a specific curriculum and methods of teaching. Another important change brought about by the new development was the formation of an association of physicians. This provided a venue for the physicians to discuss various problems, including academic as well as service matters. Last but not the least, journals were published, which did yeoman services in the areas of generation and dissemination of the knowledge of medicine.

The meaning and significance of these activities would be clear only when they are placed within their historical context. The activities of these scholar–physicians were started in a period that was vibrant with the zeal and enthusiasm of the national movement in India, the waves of which had reached every nook and corner of the subcontinent. It was in this historical context that the zealous attempts of the renaissance leaders of Āyurveda were staged in all the regions of the subcontinent. Each one mentioned in the preceding pages was a scholar and a physician who contributed richly to one or two fields of activities, such as teaching or writing books on various aspects of the science of Āyurveda.

Appendix

Auxiliary Branches of Knowledge: Treatment for Plants and Animals

Alchemy

The common man's ideas and concepts of alchemy are in the realm of legends and beliefs in notions of transmutation of base metals to precious metals, such as gold, and also in changing the internal structure of the human body. Indian alchemy is said to have two characteristic streams: gold making and elixir synthesis.[1] Stories of wonders apart, historical facts at a mundane level bear testimony to the use of some materials, such as mercury, in changing base metals to alloys of various types.

Terms such as chemistry and alchemy were made popular by the prevalence of mercury. Mercury is a metal and, at the same time, it is in a liquid form. The miraculous effects of mercury led people to believe that it is the essence extracted from all medicines. Hence it came to be designated as *rasa*, the essence. Thus, all treatments by means of minerals came to be known as *rasa* therapy.

Medicines and Elixirs

From the historical point of view, chemistry has two stages of development. The first is the study of minerals, precious

[1] A. Rahman, ed., *History of Indian Science, Technology and Culture, A.D.1000-1800* (Delhi: OUP, 1999). 152.

stones, and metals, including gold, iron, copper, diamonds, pearls, corals, and shells. The second stage is the study of mercury, sulphur, and arsenic. Indians had mastered the first stage very early; asphalt and other minerals found in some Harappan sites, which are believed to have been collected and preserved for medical use, are proof of this development. The *Ègveda* refers to the Aśvinidevas substituting the lost leg of Visphala by a thigh made of iron. Soma is one of the herbs elevated thus to divinity. It is said that the juice of this herb defeats death, hence it is called *amrita*, similar to the ambrosia of the Greeks. The invocation of soma, the elixir that removed death among the devas, deserves to be noted. The origin of chemistry can be seen in this adoration of soma juice. Similarly, invocations of other medicines can also be seen. It may be remembered here that there is a whole *sūkta* in the *Rgveda* on *oṣadhi*.[2] These hymns appear to suggest that the ideas about alchemy were prevalent in the period of the *Atharvaveda*.

Suśruta gives the medicinal properties of tin, black lead, silver, gold, and lead; Caraka also gives descriptions of five metals, except black lead. In the chapter 'Āragvadhīya', Caraka describes the medicinal properties of realgar (*manaśśila*), rock salt (*lavaṇa*), orpiment, red ochre, and so forth for skin diseases. Some scholars take the term *saugandhika* mentioned in this chapter to denote sulphur; Caraka gives a long list of minerals and artificial salts in the eighth chapter of the *Vimanasthāna* of the *Carakasamhita*; sulphur and mercury are prescribed in the treatment of leprosy. In this context, it must be remembered that Dṛḍhabala completed *Kalpasthāna*, *Siddhisthāna*, and the last 17 chapters of *Cikitsāsthāna* of the *Carakasamhita*; hence the treatment with sulphur and mercury must have been incorporated at this stage, that is, the third century CE. Suśruta has included mercury in the products from the forest; it refers to the application of ointments. Some scholars are of the opinion that this description of the application of ointments must have appeared at the time of Suśruta.[3] The use of mercury and sulphur in medical treatment was minimal in the period from Dṛḍhabala to Cakradatta and Vṛnda. Gradually, by the increase in the use of mercury and sulphur, they came to be used in the powdered form. Mercury and sulphur were known as early as Panini's time, though the medical use of them became popular only by the medieval period.

2 *Rgveda* 10: 97.

3 Valiathan, *The Legacy of Suśruta*.

Bāṇa's *Harṣacarita* gives a long list of companions and assistants of kings, including physicians, alchemists, mineralogists, priests, and so forth. Here mineralogy was an art; it was one of the 64 arts, and its aim was to make some worthy minerals out of worthless ones, that is, through alchemy; the term *jatarupaka* for gold makes this clear. Silver is said to have been produced thus.

Like Taoism in China, Indian tantrism has made invaluable contributions to medical science. The word *tantra* itself came to denote science-oriented work. The theory and practice of healing is as old as, or even anterior to, the Vedic age; it came to be designated as Āyurveda during the period of the Samhitas. Though the perception of chemistry developed after the discovery of minerals and metals and their uses for a long time, the designation as alchemy and chemistry came into being only after the appearance of mercury. The term *rasa* means fluid (*drava*); so, the general study of it is called by the name *rasaśāstra*.

The preceptors of chemistry were either *siddha*s (holy men) of the Śaiva system or Buddhists. In course of its evolution to Mahāyāna, the Buddhist religion became more inclined to tantric practices. The materialistic world view of Buddhism came to be eclipsed in this stage. Mahāyāna and Śaivism were more or less complimentary. The preceptor of *rasaśāstra* and one of the great activists of the Middle Ages was a Buddhist monk.

The *siddha*s attracted popular attention by their proclaimed supernatural powers. They claimed powers, such as keeping the fluid mercury stable by the help of fire, making silver with it, converting copper into gold, extracting oil from sulphur, melting mica in mercury, and so forth. They even claimed to fly in the air with the help of mercury pills. The word *siddha* means one who has achieved miraculous powers. (The treatment with minerals is known as *siddha vaidyam* in South India.)

There are references in Hindi literature to 84 Buddhist monks who were believed to have superhuman powers. Interestingly, there is a *siddha* character mentioned by name. Nalanda Vikramasila and Udantapura were universities that specialized in tantric studies; when they were destroyed, many *siddha*s fled to Tibet and a few to South India. Most of the tantric works that were restored were from Tibet. There were no caste distinctions among these *siddha*s. There were launderers, shoemakers, fishermen, and so forth among them. The Brahmins shunned them; however, they attracted the masses with their miracles.

Mental and Physical Accomplishments

Accomplishment (*siddhi*) is mainly two-fold, that is, *lohasiddhi* and *dehasiddhi*. *Lohasiddhi* is the state in which one accomplishes success in experiments with mercury, *rasa*, that is, the attainment of the skill to transfer the power to mercury for converting atoms of base metals into those like gold. Similarly, *dehasiddhi* is the state in which one accomplishes the skill to transfer the power to mercury for transforming old body cells into new ones. One who is endowed with such powers is called *dehasiddha*. Lohasiddhi is called mineralogy or alchemy. Dehasiddhi is achieved through the practice of lohasiddhi; in due course, this knowledge came to be confined to lohasiddhi and the aura of mystery around it was dispelled. Metallic and mineral salts used as curatives continued to be in use. The interest shifted from the illusion of making gold to the process of making its *bhasma* (ash); they remained as medicines. Chemistry in India is closely related to who was one of the 84 *siddhas*. The *siddhas* kept the knowledge a secret; so was the case of alchemy too; they did not impart it even to their progenies; they imparted this knowledge only to competent supreme authorities.

The worship of Śiva and Pārvati entangled in embrace is part of the Kauḷa system of the Śaiva cult. The *siddhas* worshipped mercury and sulphur as representing the energies of Śiva's sperm and Pārvatī's ovum respectively. The worship of mercury and sulphur thus continued for a long time among the *siddhas*.

Nāgārjuna

Tantric works such as the *Kakṣapuṭayogaśataka* and the *Tattvaprakāśika* are ascribed to Nāgārjuna. However, there is more than one person of that name—there are many Nāgārjunas in the history of Āyurveda. The work *Cittanandapatiyasi* found in the form of a manuscript at Goma Maṭha in Tibet is attributed to him.[4] Al Biruni, who visited India in the eighth century, refers to a great alchemist who lived a century before. Hsuan-tsang, who visited India in the seventh century, mentions an alchemist and scholar Nāgārjuna who lived seven or eight centuries earlier. The *Harṣacarita* refers to Nāgārjuna who

[4] Varier, *History of Āyurveda*, 195.

presented a garland, *mandākini*, to his friend, the lord of the three oceans. Thus, Nāgārjuna, a contemporary of Sātavāhana, was an alchemist, physician, and expert in *tantra*.

Mantras and Alchemy

Mercury evaporates in fire; it cannot be kept steadily even in a crucible (the liquidity and colour gave it the name quick-silver). Then, efforts were made to find out a mantra to keep it steady. In alchemy, these mantras are known as *rasankusi*. *Rasasiddhi* is the system by which one attains accomplishment (*siddhi*) by means of mantras. Some Buddhist works attribute the use of mantras in alchemy to a *siddha* by the name *Rasaṅkusa* and thus the mantric way in alchemy is called *rasaṅkusi*. The cause of the prominence of the mantras and the tantras in alchemy was that some of those who propounded the theory treated both alchemy and the mantras as equally important. These *ācāryas* who renounced everything were mendicants, truly detached from mundane life. The great preceptors, such as Bhairavanandayōgi, Bhaluki, Nandīśvara, Kambaḷi, Vyāḷi, Nāgabōdhi, and so forth, belonged to this group. The name of the preceptors mentioned by Vāgbhaṭa in Rasaratnasamuccaya, namely, Mahādēva, Bhairava, Harimahābhairava, and Śambhu lived between the period of I and II; the alchemic work, the *Ānandakanda* of Manthanabhairava, who does not appear in this list is linked with the Ceylonese Buddhist tradition. *Rasaśāstra* is described in this work in the form of questions and answers between Dēvi and Mahābhairava. Similarly, the *Rasārṇava and* the *Rudrayamalatantra* also can be attributed to a Bhairava.

The idea of rejuvenation, longevity, and immortality that become the basis of physiological alchemy can be traced back to earlier periods and sources of history. Soma of the Vedic period can be taken as a primordial form of this concept. Kautalya's *Arthaśāstra* knew the metallurgical aspects of alchemy. This text of the Mauryan period refers to the use of alchemy in making alloys, such as brass, and also in the production of other gold-like alloys. This clearly shows that the use of mercury in making gold and coloured amalgams was known at least from the Mauryan times. Several types of gold, such as *rasaviddham*, that is, one obtained by treatment with mercury, are mentioned. *Hāṭaka* also meant gold and it is an alchemical practice since it is the elixir made from mercury and other ingredients that could transmute other metals into gold.[5]

Philosophy of Mercury

Elixir or *rasāyana* is a substance that could transform other base metals into gold and silver as well as confer longevity and immortality when taken internally. In fact, gold-making was looked upon as a test to be performed prior to administering the elixir. The whole process was conceived as parallel or identical to that of culturing the human body and making it indestructible. *Rasaratnākara* says:

> I shall certainly tell you whatever is asked by you that is, remedies of warding off wrinkles and grey hair and also stop ageing. These preparations can act with equal efficacy on the metals as well as on human body.[6]

Buddhist texts of the fifth and sixth centuries CE contain recipes for synthesizing medicines from the substance of plants and mineral origin, which could give great strength and even immortality. Romila Thapar opines that alchemy developed in the early centuries of the CE, presumably when both mercury and sulphur were available and their properties familiar. The Buddhist philosopher of c. fifth century CE is described as being conversant with alchemy.[7] A Chinese source refers to an Indian taken to China by Wan Hsuan Tse in the seventh century CE. He claimed that he knew the substance for prolonging life.[8]

The early medieval period saw a considerable interest in alchemy among certain Jaina groups and later among yogi sects associated with tantrism. The fascination lay in two fundamental processes essential to alchemy—sublimation and transmutation. Through sublimation, the structure of the metal was decoded and could be changed. Transmutation was the actual changing of one metal to

[5] *Rgveda* 10: 97.

[6] Nityanatha, *Rasaratnākara*.

[7] Thapar, *Ancient Indian Social History*, 96. For a Pre-Arab date for the use of mercury in India see, P.C. Ray, *A History of Hindu Chemistry* (Calcutta, 1907–25, vol. II), 8–9.

[8] Joseph Needham, *Science and Civilization in China* (Cambridge: Needham Research Institute, 1954), 212.

another. Changing of the bodily structure is to enable the body to be transmuted to one capable of performing feats beyond the normal and for gaining new perception. Metaphorically, it was Hara and Gouri—mercury and mica—joining together to produce a new substance.

Treatment for Plants: Vṛkṣāyurveda

The medicinal value of herbs and the worship of plants have been widely known right from the beginning of the recorded histories of human cultures. In the context of Indian history, the earliest sources for this topic are the seals obtained in large numbers from the excavated sites of the Harappan civilization. Many seals from the Indus sites have motifs depicting plants and plant worship and related issues. Some of the prehistoric rock-art sites have also yielded artistic representation of the worship of plants. The *Oṣadhi Sūkta* in the tenth *maṇḍala* of the *Rgveda* is perhaps the earliest literary evidence for the medicinal value of herbs and the worship of plants wherein it is stated that the *oṣadhi* were there even prior to the gods themselves.[9] Coming to the period of recorded history, the Major Rock Edict II of the Mauryan emperor Ashoka declares that medicinal herbs were collected from places where they are available in plenty and planted them in places where they are not available—in his own territory and beyond that, in the territories of Antioch beyond the north-western boundary and in their bordering regions and also in the territories of the Cholas, Pandyas, Keralaputhras, upto the Tamraparni, that is, Ceylon. This would suggest that some method of systematic planting and growing of plants were known even at that early stage of Indian history.

The importance of herbal plants and their availability need not be reiterated in the context of the discussion on a medicinal system that is mainly based on herbal medicines. Ancient Indians were fully aware of this fact and they had developed a systematic and scientific knowledge of various aspects of plant life, including methods for culturing and growing different types of plants. What is perhaps all the more attractive is the influence of the basic concepts of the science of Āyurveda, such as the theory of *tridoṣa*, *saptadhātu*, and so forth, which are found

[9] yā oṣadhī pūrvā jātā devebhyastriyugam purā (X.97.1).

in this ancient branch of knowledge. This seems to imply that this topic of learning was, in all probability, developed with a creative inspiration from the practitioners of Āyurveda. In other words, Vṛkṣāyurveda has to be taken as an extension of the knowledge and wisdom of Āyurveda. Therefore, any meaningful discussion on Āyurveda will be complete only with reference to the topics and methods of Vṛkṣāyurveda.

According to the Ègvedic hymns, a physician is the one who possesses knowledge over thousands of medicines.[10] In the classical texts, *auṣadha* generally denotes flowers, fruits, leaves, roots, stems or other parts of creepers, trees, and other items of natural resources with the exception of some metals and minerals. The ancient sages, who were fully aware of the importance of plants for human existence, nurtured and preserved vegetation, including trees and creepers around their hermitage, with love and care. India being an agricultural country, studies on vegetation were a part of the curriculum from the very early period. In the *Atharvaveda*, the appraisal of the potentiality of plants is based on their magical effect. The study of plants had advanced considerably by the time of the classical texts, that is, the Samhitas on the basis of various aspects, such as region, season, seed, growth-pattern, and on various conditions and factors such as *tridoṣa* and *rasa* properties. However, the term Gulmavṛkṣāyurveda came to be used much later. The *Arthaśāstra* instructs rulers to preserve and maintain public parks, pleasure gardens, hunting forests, and so forth under expert supervision; the word Gulmavṛkṣāyurveda is found in this context. *Dhanvantari nighaṇṭu* defines the Vṛkṣāyurveda as the study related to the life of plants. The Vṛkṣāyurveda in its mature form is a branch of science that encompasses modern phyto-chemistry and treatments for infestations of plants. A large variety of subjects, including collection and preservation of seeds, selection of the soil, methods of sowing, and of germination, various means of grafting and cutting, planting, seedlings, nursing, manuring, cultivation during different seasons, and location of plants for improving the aesthetic and hygienic surroundings of the homestead, come under this branch of knowledge. The Buddhist literature contains a story that relates how Bhikṣu Ātreya asked his disciple Jīvaka to fetch a plant which has no medicinal properties found within an area of four square *yojanas*. This was in order to test Jīvaka's knowledge of herbal medicines. Jīvaka, naturally, came out successfully

[10] *Yatrouṣdhī samagmata rājāa vipral sa ucyate bhiṣak rakṣohāmivacātana. Ègveda*, X. 97. 3.

in the test. The essence of the story implies the high level of knowledge imparted on plant life in those days.

1. First stage—from the Vedic period to the Gupta period (600 CE)
2. Second stage—from 601 to 1536, and
3. Third stage—from 1536 onwards.

Vedic Times upto the Gupta Period (600 CE)

The period witnessed major historical events, including the eastward migration of the Vedic people and the unprecedented large-scale human settlements in the Ganga–Yamuna doab. People must have come in contact with a large number of plants, creepers, and trees. It is only logical to think that there were attempts on the part of the learned people to gather knowledge about the vegetation in their surroundings. It can be learnt from the later Vedic texts, including the Brāhmaṇas, the *Āraṇyakas*, and the *Upaniṣads*, that the knowledge of geographical regions in the Āryāvartta as well as various aspects of vegetation was acquired and preserved by the time of these texts. Significantly enough, the entire universe was viewed by the great sages of this age as an *aśvattha* tree (*Ficus religiosa*) with its roots upwards and branches leaning downwards.

One of the topics of interest in this period was the knowledge of various types of plants. The accumulation of information in this aspect resulted in various methods of classification of plants into various sections, such as *vriksha, gulma, śāka, vīrudh, stabaka,* and so forth. Another mode of classification was on the basis of their varied reproductive ways, such as those born from seeds (*bījaruha*), those from roots (*mulajam*), those from stem (*skandajam*), those spread in stem (*skandaropaniyam*), those sprouting from leaves (*parnayoni*) in works such as the *Bṛhatsamhita*, the *Arthaśāstra*, the *Manusamhita*, and so forth. The classification was also based on their properties, characteristics, morphological specialities, regional links, surroundings, and so on. For example, based on the properties, some are classified into *vānīra, dantadhāvana, lekhana,* and *kārpāsa,* which indicates their use in day-to-day life. Those having medicinal properties are referred to as *dadrughna, arśoghna, śōphani,* and so forth. *Phēnila, bahupada, carmina,* and others, are according to their peculiarities. Some names denote their morphological specialities—for example, *tripatra, kesaparṇi, pancāṅgula, hemapushpa, satamuli*, and *sataparṇika*. Based on regional connections, a few are classified as *sauvira*, *camabaya*, *magadhi*, *orapushpa*, and others. Some terms remind us of their surroundings, such as *nadisarja*, *jalaja*, *maruvaka*, and so on. Names such as *bakuḷa*, *śītabhīru*, *maghya*, and *śarada* show various other peculiarities. Plants have common as well as medicinal names. The former are identification names, while the latter indicate their properties; for example, *citrabīja* and *vatari* are synonyms. *Ricinus communis*, *vakrapuṣpa*, and *vrajari* are other names of *jayanti* (*Premna corymbosa*). The mode of classification is divided into three types, namely, botanical (*udbhitam*), medicinal (*virecana*), and dietetic (*a<u>n</u>napā<u>n</u>am*). Botanically, a tree that brings forth fruits without flowering is known as *vanaspati*, one that bears flowers and fruits is called a *vṛkṣa*, and those that exist as annual crops are called *auṣadhi*. Among vines, those that crawl along the ground are called *pratanini*, and those that climb around trees are *valli*. Small plants with juicy stems are *gulma*, while those belonging to the grass and bamboos are called *tṛṇadhvaja*, *avatana*, and *druma*. Another classification was on the basis of medical science. Caraka divides plants into two groups, that is, *kaṣāyas* (decoctions) and *virecanas* (purgatives); *kaṣāyas* are 500 and *virecanas* are 600 in number. The *kaṣāyas* are segregated into 10 varieties and groups; each group consists of 50 items. Suśruta has divided them into 37 groups and all the medicinal herbs that were known in that period are included in these groups. Division is also made on their dietetic use. Caraka divides them into six groups, namely, grains, pulses, vegetables, fruits, Hārīta (such as ginger, lime, onions, garlic), edible oils, and *ikṣus* (such as sugarcane). The classification is more detailed and systematic in the *Suśrutasamhita*. It classifies medicinal herbs into 15 groups, namely *śāli*, *vrīhi*, *kudhānya*, *śamidhānya*, *vaidala*, *tila*, *yava*, *simbava* and its variations, *phala*, *śāka*, *puṣpa*, *udbhida*, *kanda*, *taila*, and *ikṣu*. Creepers and climbing plants are fragile; they are classified into two—those that twine and creep over a tree, and those that spread on the ground. Those that do not harm the tree are called *vrkṣaruha* (epiphytes); those like parasites are *vṛkṣādani*; lichen is called *jalanīlika* and mushrooms are *catra*; and mosses are called *śaivala*.

Plant diseases

The *Atharvaveda* contains studies on plant diseases; it also mentions plant pests. Commenting on this, Sayana gives a long list of such pests. The works of Vinaya contain studies on blotting of seeds and fungus; there are descriptions in the *Śukranīti* on crop damage from poison, fire, frost, and insects. One chapter each of the *Arthaśāstra* and the *Bṛhadsamhita* is on Vṛkṣāyurveda. The *Bṛhadsamhita* describes the prognosis and treatments of plant diseases. Futility or infertility of plants was considered as a disease; a whole chapter in the *Śārṅgadharapaddhati* entitled 'Upavanavinoda' is devoted to this topic. Buddhist texts such as the *Vinayapiṭaka* contain useful information about the diseases affecting sugarcane and grains.

The next stage in this branch of knowledge may be described as morphology of plants, that is, the descriptive accounts of different parts of plants. Later Vedic texts, such as the *Taittiriyasamhita* and the *Vājasaneyasamhita*, dilate on various parts of plants. Thus, the plant has the *mūla* (root) and the *tūla* (shoot). The tūla consists of the stem, branch, flower, and fruit; the trees have a trunk, branch, and leaves. Interestingly, there is a portion in the *Śukrānīti* that metaphorically compares the king of a country, its councillors, commanders, troops, subjects, and the land to the various parts of trees, such as roots, stems, branches, leaves and flowers, fruits, and seeds.[11] What is significant in this is the reference to various aspects and functions of the state help us to place the text in its historical setting. The process of state formation in ancient India is attributed after consulting various sources of information, including excavated materials and literary texts to the middle of the first millennium BCE.[12]

According to Suśruta, germination occurs only when the season, soil, and water are combined in the proper order. The seed sprouts by bursting the outer skin of the seed. India had known from the early date as suggested by various sources that the appropriate combination of vāta, pitta, and kapha (air, warmth, and water) are required for germination. The term *uttānapāda* significantly denotes that it is the *pāda* or the root that comes out first during germination; mūla is the term for the base and root. When the roots decay, the branches wither away and the tree perishes. *Pādapa*, the synonym for tree, meaning that which drinks with the foot, indicates that it is the roots that absorb

[11] This text is referred to in the *Arthaśāstra* of Kautalya, thereby implying that the work is pre-Mauryan.

[12] R.S. Sharma, *Material Culture*, 166.

the liquid food; spreading roots are called *śākhāśiphas* and fibrous roots *śiphas* or *jaṭas*.

The trunk of a tree named tūla or *vistāra* has two parts: stem as well as leaves; the stem may be with internodes and nodes from where leaves sprout; a stem without branches or candex is called *sthāṇu* or *śaṅku*. A bush is called *kṣupa*. Branches are described as *aṉuśākhas*, *pratiśākhas*, and *ausākhas* in the descending order of their size. The underground portion, which looks like roots, are called *kanda*. They may be tubers (as in the case of yam) or bulbs (as in the case of onions), and are the means of reproduction. The bud is called *pravāḷa*. Leaves are called *patras* as that which fall easily, and *parṇas* due to the green colour. It may be *savṛnda* (petiolate) or *avṛnda* (sessile); the number of leaves in a cluster may be equal, that is, *ēkapatra* (unifoliate), or *dvipatra*, or *tripatra*, or *saptapatra*, and so forth, according to their nature. Plants are often named according to the shape of their leaves, such as *aśvakarṇika* (horse's ear), *mūṣikaparṇi* (rat-leaved), *keśaparṇi* (hair-leaved), *hamsapadi* (swan-footed), and so on.

The modern taxonomy based on natural classification of species with their family analysis was not known then. However, plants having similar qualities and characters were grouped together. The *kōvidāra* group encompasses the white, yellow, and red varieties; the white varieties were again subdivided into two. There were four varieties of *bala*, that is, *bala*, *atibala*, *mahābala*, and *nāgabala*.

The propriety and accuracy shown by the authorities in understanding and describing different parts of plants and various asects of them are admirable. The names in most cases are not simply names alone but they carry an element of analytical thinking. Flowers are *prasūna* and *sumanas*. The buds not fully opened are called *kalika* or *kōraka* and at the blooming stage it is *mukuḷa* or *kuḍmaḷa*; when fully opened, they are *vikaca* or *sphuṭa*. A bunch of flowers arranged as cymose is called *stabaka* or *gucchaka* and as racemose is called *matjari*. The terms like *śrīhastini* and *chatra* denote a kind of floral decoration. The stalk of a flower is called *prasavabandhini*, that which joins flowers and fruits to the mother tree. The *puṣpacchada* (calyx), *dala* (petal), *kēsara* (stamens), *parāga*, and *kesarareṇu* (pollen) are parts of the flower; since the term differentiating gynoecium (*garbhakesaras*) with the male androecium is not found, it is assumed that it was not studied in that period. But some species such as *tala* (*Borassus flabellifer*) were found divided as male and female.

The fruit is significantly called *phala*, suggesting that it indicates the result of a long process of transformation in the previous stages. The fruits are termed by different names, that is, green fruits as *śalasu*, fleshy one as *jalaka* or *kshīraka*, dry-fruits as *vana*, and legume kinds as *simbi*; often they are named after the nature of their mother tree—for instance *āmra*, *jambu*, *aiṅguda*, *vainavadi*, and so forth. The *bīja*, meaning seed, is the base of a plant; its pericarp is *bījakośa*, the kernel or endosperm is *sasya*, and the cotyledon is *bijapatra* or *bijadala*. The *Śārṅgadharaparampara* exquisitely describes the complete development stage of a mango tree.

The internal morphology of plants could not have been properly observed before the invention of a microscope. Ancient Indians had identified five parts in plants, that is, the bark (*tvak*), soft tissues (*māmsa*), bone or wood (*asthi*), pith (*majja*), and fibres (*snāyu*). The *Bṛhadāraṇyaka* divides the *māmsa* portion into two—the covering (*valkala*) and the fibre portion (*sakara*). There is a reference to the natural healing (*ropaṇa*) in plants in the commentary of the *Guṇaratna* and in the appendix of the Śaṅkaramitra.

Indians had found out, probably from an early date, though not in the modern scientific manner, that trees absorb food in the liquid form from the soil and it is taken to the leaves through the trunk and branches; the leaves transform it to food with the help of air and the sun. It is on account of this metabolic process that plants grow. The *Vaiseṣika* of *Kaṇāda* and the *Upaskara* of *Śaṅkaramitra* discuss processes of the water being poured at the base of a tree that reaches all its parts. Nature (*niyati*) is its cause; the unseen being instrumental and water, the material causes.

Rajanighaṇṭu explains the process of the exudation of sap in plants; the phenomenon of phosphorrescence in plants is also noted; such illuminating plants are called *jyotiṣmati*, *jyotirlata*, and so on.

Vedic texts, the Itihāsa–Purāṇa tradition, and the ancient and medieval literature, including original works and commentaries, have observed the world of plants and recorded facts that are valid even today. From the Vedic age, Indians have observed that plants have life. Different phases of life, such as childhood, youth, and old age, are seen in plants too. The development of life is governed by the nourishment provided by light, food, and water. The maximum life of a plant is calculated to be 10,000 years. Plants seek favourable conditions. Their leaves fold up when they sleep at night; some are sensitive to touch; some others blossom at different times. The ancient people had keenly observed all these characteristics. Manu observes that plants have an intuitive power to feel joy and sorrow. The santiparva of the Mahabharata, *Bhgavatapurāṇa*, the commentary of Guṇaratna, Kiraṇāvali of Udayana, the appendix in Kanada—all contain discussions on the life of plants. In those days, the people had a good knowledge regarding the reproductive system of plants.

Though there is no scrupulous knowledge on their gender variation, references are made to plants such as *tala* and *ketaki* having gender variations. For instance, the fruitless ketaki belongs to the male gender known as *silaketaki*, and that which bears fruits, the female gender, is known as *svarnaketaki*. Ecology was also important. The studies in Āyurvedic works on the classification of land as *jāṅgala* (dry), *anūpa* (marshy), *and sadharana* (ordinary) are very specific. Taxonomy had made much progress in the very early period. Sir William Jones opines that Mr Linnieaus would have accepted this classification if only he had studied the old language. Names such as *bodhidruma*, *aśoka*, *Śivaśekhara*, and *yajṭadruma* are some examples of grouping according to special characteristics.

According to an early concept, plants are the lowest living form of evolution. In the *Taittiriya Upanishad*, the description of the order of evolution is: the sky (ether) from the soul, from ether the air, from air the fire, from fire the water, from water the earth, from earth the plants, and from plants the human beings. The discussion on heredity in Caraka is well known.

The *Śārṅgadharapaddhati* and *Bṛhadsamhita* describe artificial means to produce potential herbs so also to give fragrance to flowers. Cotton was produced in red, yellow, and blue colours from a very early period. The growth of plants determined the market price; the price was also speculated. Plant growth was taken as a standard to assess the sumptuous presence of ground water. Medical science, agriculture, horticulture, and forestry all are allied to plants. There is an ancient work by the name *Krishisaṅgraha*. Many sayings attributed to Vana are still relevant. The rotation of crops was practised even in Rgvedic times.

Medieval Period

Systematic studies on phyto-chemistry developed during this period. The significant contribution of this period was the work *Upavanavinoda* of Śārṅgadhara (1283–1301) who adorned the court of the king

Hammira. The text contains various subjects such as taxonomy, selection of seeds, sowing, transplantation, irrigation, protection, treatment, propagation, and so forth.

Modern Period

The modern period has two phases—the first from 1563 to 1848 CE and the rest, the second. The systematic study in phyto-chemistry developed in this era. This era started with the publication of *Coloquios Dos Simples E drogas Da India*, a work on medicinal plants by Gracia Da Orta (1563). Many scholars followed him. Another work of scientific importance is *Hortus Malabaricus* by Henry Van Reed, the then Dutch governor of Malabar. John Gerard Koenig, the Danish phyto-chemist, who reached India in 1768 set up a society by the name United Brothers in Tran Queue Bar in association with Hayne, Clain, and Rottler. They encouraged the study of particular plants in isolation and also in exchange with that of Europe. Many stalwarts of the time associated themselves with the United Brothers. It played a creative role in this field for a long time; the French in Pondicherry enriched them later.

Lieutenant Colonel Robert Kyid set up a Royal Botanical Gardens in 1787 at Calcutta. He was its first superintendent. Its aim, though monetary, was to cultivate teak and Malayan spices. However, later it was transformed into the first recognized centre for botanical activities. Roxburgh (1751–1815) who succeeded Kyid entitled for the name of Indian Linnieus. Following him, many renowned scientists toured Nepal, South India, and other regions, identified the plants and brought out illustrated publications on about 2,500 plants. They worked in union with famous European scientists. The contribution of Griffith who travelled through the Assam valley, Burma, Bhutan, Sikkim, central India, Korasan and Malacca, and collected about 9,000 species is remarkable. Many valuable publications followed in this era. A second botanical centre was started at Sahranpur in 1820. Many eminent scientists had associated themselves with this centre. In general, many scientists from the West worked in this field and brought out several publications.

The second phase starts with the activities of Sir Joseph Hooker, in association with his friend Thomas Thomson. The remarkable discoveries of Rhododendron species were during this stage. His work, *The Flora of British India*, has been published in seven volumes.

Thomas Anderson exerted to cultivate the plant cinchona, the source of quinine. The marked feature of this phase was the setting up of the Indian Forest Department. Lindsay Stewart, Colonel Beddome, Sir D. Brandis, and Messers Talbot and Gamble, all had contributed much to develop a methodical study of Indian phyto-chemistry. The first Indian writer in this field was Upendralal Kancilal; his work, *Flora of Assam*, was completed by his son P.C. Kancilal.

Many European scientists conducted studies and research in the Madras presidency. A second public herbarium was established in Madras with the efforts of Bedie and Lawson. The Botanical Survey was founded in 1890; its publication, *Annals of the Royal Botanic Gardens*, brought out the studies of important species and genera of Indian plants with due importance. They took interest in profitably cultivating cash crops, such as tea, cinchona, rubber, and so forth. In 1883, a department came into being to manage all the profit-making entities of the Indian empire. The *Dictionary of Economic Products* by George Watts was a remarkable work of this phase. The Forest Department commenced systemic works and modalities from 1847; gradually forest colleges came up at Cooper Hill and Dehradun. The official journals of the Bengal Asiatic Society (1784) and the Bombay Natural History Society brought out research articles in botany for over a century.

Even though universities came up in a few provinces in the nineteenth century, botanical studies in these educational centres were started only in the first decade of the twentieth century. Bengal started botanical studies with the establishment of a medical college in 1835. The first Indian who produced a botanical work in his vernacular language was Yadugopal Mukherji in 1869. In the post-renaissance period, the inquisitive youth showed much interest in botanical studies too. About 1,510 key papers came out in botanical studies between 1868–1911; of these, 34 were by Indians. In 1914, the Indian Science Congress was established and the Indian Botanical Society was set up in 1920. The Bose Research Institute in the name of J.C. Bose was founded in 1917. Today, facilities for the study of botany are available in all Indian universities; many research papers come out every year.

Life in plants

There is an *ākāśa* (ether) predominance even in the hardest woods for they also yield fruits and flowers (V1); The barks, fruits, and flowers wither away in the heat; they possess a sense of touch (V2); fruits and flowers are shattered down by the wind, thunder, and lighting; they possess a sense of hearing (V3); manuring, medicated watering, and fumigating cures plant infestation and bloom again; they possess the sense of smell (V4); they suck water by roots (as by the mouth), succumb to ailments for lack of watering, and get cured by treatment; they possess the sense of taste (V5). They discern glee and gloom, and though cut-off, shoot-forth; they have life (V6); the life enables them to absorb water, light, and air; they possess the power of assimilation and self-nutrition (V7).

Veterinary Science: Treatment for Animals

It is necessary to have at least a primary knowledge of the role played by various animals such as cattle, horses, and elephants in the ancient Indian economy, society, and and culture in order to understand the relevance of a subject such as Aśvāyurveda. The Allchins have maintained that the wild species of horse appeared in the late Pleistocene times on the south Russian and Ukranian steppes, and then eastwards towards Khazakstan and Central Asia and also, therefore, domestication of it took place in those regions sometime before 2000 BCE.[13] This means that the animals' natural habitat was a region of low humidity. The Allchins furnish interesting information that the Boghazkeui inscription mentions details of horse-training by Kikkuli of Mitanni using chariot-racing terms in virtually pure Sanskrit. The term *aśva*, meaning horse, is used several times in its various forms in the hymns of the *Rgveda*.[14] It has been calculated that 'there are over fifty five personalities with horse-connected names and thirty with chariot connected names in vedic literature'.[15] Recently, there is a sudden augment of interest in the species following a search for the nativity of the Vedic people and this has resulted in a debate on the date of early occurrences of the horse in India.

[13] Bridget Allchin and Raymond Allchin, *The Birth of Indian Civilization* (Harmondsworth, England: Penguin Books, 1968), 144.

[14] R.S. Sharma, *Material Culture*, 22–3, *passim*.

[15] Edwin Bryant, *The Quest for the Origins of the Vedic Culture* (New Delhi: Oxford University Press 2002), 170.

Aśvāyurveda: Treatment for Horses

There is a considerable amount of literature pertaining to the various topics of protection and treatment of animals, especially horses and elephants. This is quite understandable in the context of various historical developments on the subcontinent, including the advent of the Aryan-speaking people to the north-western parts of the subcontinent with the horse as their efficient riding animal of speed and strength, their characteristic agni ritual, their spread to the eastern parts up to the eastern places of the Ganga–Yamuna Doab, an unprecedented increase in agricultural production, the proliferation of urban centres well connected by trade routes, the formation of a state based on the income from these sources, the presence of mutually conflicting royal houses, and so on. The use of animals was well known, especially on trade routes as pack animals and on war fronts as fighting animals.

A plausible piece of archaeological evidence from a superficial level of Mohenjo-Daro for the presence of horse has already been mentioned.[16] Horses belong to different varieties, such as Equus *caballus* Linn, Equus *asinus*, Equus *Hemionus khur*, and so forth.[17] The presence of a genuine horse Equus *caballus* at Hallur in the beginning of the Neolithic-chalcolithic phase is dated to 1400–1050 BCE. Several sites, including Bagor in Rajasthan, at the base of the Aravalli hills, and the Neolithic site at Hallur in Karnataka, have been suggested with the remains of the horse. *Uttarāpatha*, the ancient Eastern Highway, the one connecting the Ganga–Yamuna valleys with the north-western countries, such as Gandhāra, Kambōja, and so forth, was famous as the route of a fine breed of horses. Horse dealers from the western regions traded with the eastern Indian cities, such as Kāśi (Benaras), Pāṭalīputra (Patna), Prāgjyōtiṣapura (Assam), and so forth. These north-western traders established contacts not only with the regions on the subcontinent but also with Myanmar, south-western China, South-East Asian regions, and even upto Sri Lanka. The Chinese envoy Chiang Kien is said to have seen in Gāndhāra in circa 127 BCE bamboo and textiles from south-western China. What we would conclude on these evidences is that the horse was an important animal that was present on the subcontinent at least from the date of the Vedic people with different functions in economic, social, and

[16] Allchin and Allchin, *The Birth of Indian Civilization*, 260.

[17] Medow, 1987, 909.

cultural aspects of life. This seems to account for the interest in the well-being of the animal and the presence of a fairly good amount of literature in this branch of knowledge. It may be noted in this connection that some works that appeared at an early date dealing with the treatment for horses refer to the mobilization of cavalry in various orders.[18]

In those days, numerous routes traversed the subcontinent, some continuing further into central and western Asia. The political control of the Śakas and Kuṣāṇas linked Central-Asian regions with India. Once the connection had been established, trade would continue provided there were enough goods available for exchange. Chinese traders imported fur and horses and so horse trade was also of considerable interest to Indian traders.[19]

Some sort of diversification in trading activities due to specialization in trade has been noted as an important development in contemporary South Indian trades.[20] There are innumerable references in the Coḷa inscriptions of the thirteenth and fourteenth centuries to a special group of horse-dealers, the Kutiraicceṭṭis, who are said to be hailing from Malaimaṇḍalam, namely Kerala.[21] They figure prominently in the inscriptions of Tanjavur, Tiruccirappalli, and South Arcot districts. Apparently, they imported horses from foreign countries, such as Arabia and Tegu, and supplied them to the princes and nobles of South India.[22] Interestingly, horse trade is mentioned as a lucrative business for Kerala merchants in a Malayalam literary text of this period.[23] A spurt in horse trade in these parts of the country is partly explained by the political developments in the South Indian territories, which were constantly engaged in quarrels among the regional

18 *Salihothram, Uttarottarasthanam.*

19 Romila Thapar, *Early India from the Origins to AD 1300* (London : Penguin, 2002), 235.

20 R. Champakalakshmi, *Urbanisation in South India: The Role of Ideology and Polity* (Presidential address, Section I: Ancient India, Indian History Congress, 47th Session, Srinagar, 1986), 21.

21 See *ARISE* 201 of 1905; 161 of 1907; 59, 346, 361, 393, 399, 429, 503, 537, and 538 of 1919; 182 of 1926; 196 of 1927–8; 15, 16 of 1935–6; 34, 50, and 77 of 1936–7.

22 Nilakanta Sastri, *The Colas* (Madras University, 1984 (1935–7)), 607. See also T.V. Mahalingarn, *South Indian Polity*, 388.

23 *Unniyaccicaritam* (Kottayam: Sahityapravarthaka Co-operative Society, 2002), 18, stanza 78.

and local powers.[24] The rulers of local principalities in Kerala also maintained a cavalry as alluded to by some literary texts.[25]

Wasaf, a Persian historian, informs us that the price of each horse was fixed at 220 dinar of red gold (equal to 440 seggi of Marco Polo) on the condition that if any horse should happen to die, their value should be paid from the royal treasury.[26] Wasaf gives the total number and the value of the annual import of horse trade as 10,000 animals worth 22 lakhs of dinars of red gold. According to the same author, the imported horses that are strong, swift, fresh, and active become weak, slow, useless, and stupid within a short time due to the wrong type of feeding and other treatment. Hence, there was the necessity of importing new horses annually. Marco Polo also was of the same opinion that the people of South India did not know how to take care of horses.[27] A large amount of wealth acquired by those who were involved in the profitable long-distance overland trade is reflected in their donations in the form of structural buildings, large number of cattle, landed property, and big amount of money to the distant regional centres of worship.

Veterinary Science and Horticulture in Ancient India

Scholars are of the opinion that the accomplishments of Indians in veterinary science in the ancient period can be considered on par with the knowledge of Europeans in the nineteenth century. The beginning of the Indian tradition of veterinary science is generally traced to the *Atharvaveda*. A sedative prescribed against the germs that infest animals is seen in one of the hymns (ii: 32). Remedies are also prescribed for parasitic diseases in cattle. Jaina literature contains accounts of the world of plants and the similarities and dissimilarities of the life cycles of human beings and plants. Sophisticated women of that time are said to have been well versed in many branches of

[24] For the political history of South India during the period under discussion, see Nilakanta Sastri, *A History of South India* (3rd edn.) (Oxford University Press, 1971 [1966]), the chapter on 'The Age of the Four Kingdoms', 211–24.

[25] *Unnunilisandesam* (Kottayam: Sahityapravarthaka Co-operative Society, 2014), 1, 60.

[26] Elliot and Dowsen, *A History of India According to their Historians*, Vol. III (1871 edn.), 34.

[27] K.D. Swarninathan, 'The Horse Traders of Malai-mandalam', *Journal of Indian History*, 1954, 32(2): 138–43.

knowledge, including the knowledge of treatment and training of horses, rearing of elephants, medical science, chemistry and plant care. According to one authority, horticulture was one among the 64 arts in which they had to gain proficiency. Megasthanese and Arrian praise the ability of Indians in driving chariot in circles. Treating the animals was always a practical need, and so there were veterinary physicians everywhere. The *smritis* testify to the scientific system of treatments for animals that prevailed here from very early times. *Manusmṛti* speaks of public grazing land for cattles. The *Parāśarasamhita* observes that if a cow succumbs to death during treatment in spite of all precautions, no compensation was to be paid; but atonement was called for if it dies for want of care; similar description are there in the *Dharmaśāstra* texts of Āpastamba and Samvṛtta too. It is learnt from these works that the blood test was made to decide the nature of death after the death of cattle; this seems to indicate a system of postmortem examination. However, there are no references to such a system in the case of humans in any of the medical or ethical texts. The *Arthaśāstra* of Kautalya speaks of *āśumṛtaka parīkṣa*, that is, a system of investigation of sudden death in the context of crime and punishment in the chapter on *Kaṇṭakaśōdhana*, literally, removing thorns. Dead bodies of the victims of hanging, drowning, and poisoning were kept in special rooms; such rooms, similar to the mortuaries of modern times, were set up in all districts throughout the empire. We hear from the same source that oils were used to preserve dead bodies.

Aśvāyurveda

The treatment of horses and elephants, and the protection of cows, trees, and plants had developed along with Āyurveda from very ancient times. There was knowledge regarding the physiology of animals from the Vedic period onwards. Each and every internal and external organ was named and their functions observed. Physicians had to study the physiology of animals and we have already noted (in Chapter 2, 'Monastic Knowledge of Anatomy') that this was perhaps the beginning of the knowledge of anatomy in India. The most celebrated text in veterinary science is *Sālihōtram* named after Sālihotra, the author of the text. The legends claim that Sālihōtra learnt Aśvāyurveda directly from Brahma and specialized in that branch of science.

Sālihōtra

Sālihōtra finds mention in some sources as the son of Hayaghōṣa and the father of Suśruta. The work *Sālihōtram* is in the form of replies to the questions of his son on Aśvāyurveda.[28] This work discusses all aspects of equestrianism and its related subjects, such as history, types, uses, controlling, training, nourishment, stabling, grazing, and so forth, hence it is considered an authoritative work. Even the job pertaining to this was named as Sālihōtram; the veterinary physicians of north-western states were known as *sāluttar*, perhaps a derived term from *Sālihōtram*. The work *Sālihōtram*, which discusses the subject elaborately, has eight *sthānas*, parts, and each of them is divided into many chapters.

NATIVITY OF SĀLIHŌTRA Sālīhōtra belonged to Sālātu of Gandhara, modern Kandahar. Some opine that he is Panini, while some others believe that he is Dhanvantari. Many scholars do not support the view of Cunningham that the place Salatu is present-day Lahore. According to Hsuan-tsang, the place called Salatulo is six *li* (Chinese mile) away to the north-west of Ohinda; this goes with the birthplace Sālātura of Pāṇini who is also called Sālātureeya. The term Sālātura denotes this place in the copper plate inscriptions of the Vallabhis of Kathiawar. According to Nakula, Sālihōtra was the son of Hayaghoṣa or Turaṅga-ghōṣa, a Brahmin who hailed from Śrāvasti. He imparted the science to his disciples at his hermitage in the Campakavāsi jungle of Magadha.

CONTENTS OF *SĀLIHŌTRAM* In the preface of the work, Suśruta requests Sālihōtra to describe the origin of horses and their treatments. Sālihōtra addresses Suśruta as 'son' and explains the story of horses. The science that he learned from Brahma consisted of 100,025 verses, which Sālihōtra abridged to eight portions and 18,000 verses. The eight *sthānas* or chapters of this work are *Unnayasthāna*, *Uttarasthāna*, *Sareerikasthāna*, *Cikitsasthāna*, *Asubhaishajyasthāna*, *Uttarottarasthāna*, *Siddhisthāna*, and *Rahasyasthāana*. Of these, only the *Unnayanasthāna* is available now, that too in a mutilated from; all the portions are available in the manuscript library of Baroda.

The first chapter of the *Unnayanasthāna* dilates on the origin of Āyurveda and refers to the treatment for horses. The second chapter,

[28] See Chapter 2, 'Monastic Knowledge of Anatomy'.

'Vidyādhyayana', describes the terms of initiation of disciples. The *Unnayanasthāna* deals with a wide range of subjects, such as types of horses, pregnancy and its course, colours of horses, four varieties, signs, natures, curls on the body, age, gait, odours, and so forth, four kinds of autumn diseases that create difficulty in the intake of water, studies on height, girth and family, various conditions in healthy and unhealthy animals, study of 10 organs, points to be noted when buying horses, taming of the wild horses, and so forth.

The first chapter, reasonably entitled *Mahāpraśna*, in the *Uttarasthāna* raises various queries. The next 39 chapters deal with a number of diseases, symptoms, and their treatments. In the third chapter *Śārīrikasthāna*, subjects such as the formation of the embryo, structure of the parts of body, development of foetus, blood vessels, nerves, the favourable environments as per the places, horses of low standard, construction of water reservoir with stones, deaf, dumb, and blind horses, shoulder diseases, study of various types of grasses, swelling wounds due to external and internal causes, obstruction of urine, fistula treatment, cancer treatment, treatment for facial paralysis, vaginal defects, seminal defects, signs of mare, and so forth are discussed.

Different types of diseases and their treatments are discussed in the *Cikitsāsthāna*. A chapter named *Miśraka* is on miscellaneous diseases such as various fevers, skin diseases, worms in the bowels, and fractures.

The *Uttarōttarasthāna* is appended to the main text. It contains instructions for building the stable, and makes mentions of several rituals and magico-religious acts, such as *rēvantapūja*, *Lakṣmīpūja*, and so forth. It also discusses the influence of asterism of *svati* and so forth, and some systems such as *nīrājanakriya* and *lohādiharana*, studies on the movements of horses.

The *Siddhisthāna* deals with mishaps arising from the improper administration of oils, milk, wines, grains, salts, and so forth, and the difficulties caused by the improper use of instruments, such as *nadi* for enema and so forth.

The eighth part, the *Rahasyasthāna*, with 24 chapters, studies the stripes on horses, that is, of their positions, importance, the longevity, symptoms of approaching death, and so forth. Various medical preparations, such as *haritakikalpa*, *rasonakalpa*, *guggulukalpa*, *lākṣākalpa*, *triphalākalpa*, *svarjikakalpa*, and treatments, such as *rasāyana* and *vājīkaraṇa*, are also dealt with. Other topics discussed in these chapters include taming and training of horses, using horses as draught animals, mobilization of cavalry in various orders, harnessing on chariots, management of stables, chanting of magical hymns, and preventive remedial measures.

Sālihotrōnnaya

The work *Sālihotrōnnaya* is written in the form of a conversation between Sālihōtra and Suśruta. Some recent scholars are of the opinion that it appears to be a comparatively recent work presented in the old style.[29] The first three chapters are legends and the remaining chapters deal with general subjects such as age, colour, qualities, marks, and so forth of the horses. Most of its chapters seem to have been lost.

Suśruta in Sālihōtram

In *Sālihōtram*, Suśruta is described as the son of Sālihōtra. Is this Suśruta the author of the *Suśrutasamhita*? According to *Suśrutasamhita*, Suśruta is the son of Viśvāmithra; Aṉuśāsanaparva of the Mahābhārata also refers to him as the son of Viśvāmitra. This leads to some confusion. Many scholars opine that as the preceptors used to address the disciples as 'sons', Suśruta could be a disciple of Sālihōtra. The reference to Ātreya in the *Hārītasamhita* addressing his disciple Hārīta as 'son' supports this view. The name of Suśruta appears in the *Aśvacikitsa* of Nakula and in the *Asvavaidya* of Jayadatta as the disciple of Sālihōtra. Jayadatta quotes Sālihōtra, Nakula, Śārṅgadhara, and Jayadeva. Gaṇa states that his work, *Aśvāyurveda*, is based on Sālihōtram; he does not mention Suśruta. He points out in the concluding portion that the work is a combilation of Sālihōtra, Suśruta, and Gārga. It can be seen that Pālakāpya and Sālihōtra are quoted as the early authoritative narrators of veterinary science in the early works; their names are referred to in the *Tattvacandrika*, a commentary to Cakradatta, of Śivadāsa Sen, but does not mention Suśruta. The *Agnipurāṇa* says that Suśruta learnt the treatment of horses, elephants, and cattle from Dhanvantari. The Bower manuscript refers to Suśruta who requests the sage Kāśirāja to explain the properties of garlic. Thus, Suśruta is mentioned as proficient in many branches of medicine, but the reference to him as the son of Sālihōtra appears only in this work.

[29] Varier, *History of Āyurveda*, 233.

Aśvapraśamsa *and* Aśvalakṣaṇaśāstra

These two works are also ascribed to Sālihōtra. The work *Aśvapraśamsa* is a small treatise in the form of lessons being imparted to Suśruta by Salihothra. *Aśvalakṣaṇaśāstra* is a study on different types of domesticated horses. The characteristic features of ideal horses, their longevity, vital points, tending, and so forth are described in this. This work refers to *Aśvaśāstrasamudra* of Simhadatta.

Later Works

Gārga is another author of *Aśvāyurveda*. Quotations from Gārga can be seen in the work of Gaṇa, though his work is not available now. The *Nītisāra* of Śukrācārya gives an elaborate description of the subject. *Asvavid* (knower of horses) is one of the titles of King Naḷa. According to the Mahabharata, Drona taught the art of the training of horses to Nakula and that of cattle to Sahadēva. Reference has been made in the *Aśvalakṣaṇaśāstra* to a work, *Aśvaśāstrasamudra*, of Simhadatta. Another notable name in the treatment of horses is the sage Vātsya. Jayadeva is an author who is often quoted by Jayadatta. The *Hayalīlāvati* is still another work; Mallīnātha Śāstri quotes verses from this work. Bhoja, the famous scholar-king of Dhārānagara, has composed a work on this science but the text is not available; In *Yuktikalpataru*, Bhoja refers to load-carrying and other animals. Another work, the *Aśvavaidyaśāstra*, is of Dīpāṅkura. The description of horses appears in the *Kavikalpalata*; The *Turaṅgaparīkṣa* of Vasantarāja is another work, which deals with the physiognomical characteristics of horses. The *Śārṅgadhara* and the *Vājicikitsa* are two other works authored by Śārṅgadhara. Indrasēna has composed a work entitled the *Sārasaṅgraha* in 1812 based on Sālihōtra. The work *Mānapriyamata* deals with the qualities of horses and the method of calculating their age. This fairly long list shows that the subject had attracted scholarly interest right from the period of the epic Mahabharata through the medieval centuries upto the modern periods.

Hayaghōṣa and Aśvaghōṣa

It is believed that Aśvaghōṣa was a contemporary of the Kuṣāṇa king Kaniṣka and was connected with the ancient city of Puruṣapura, modern Peshawar. He lived in the initial centuries CE, and was a Brahmin who hailed from Sākēta, and later became a Buddhist. According to some other sources, Hayaghōṣa was a Brahmin who spent his life in the Himalayan foothills. Sālihōtra, who imparted the science of horses to Suśruta, was much earlier to the period of Kaniṣka. All these underscore that Hayaghosha, the father of Sālihōtra and Asvaghoṣa, a contemporary of Kaniṣka, could not be the same person.

Instead of partaking in the never-ending controversies about the identity of the authors and their works, it is safe and fruitful to rely confidently on the available text to cull out the maximum valuable data pertaining to the growth of the science of Aśvāyurveda. If we look at the issue from this angle, we come across some influential works that were translated into several Indian and foreign languages. As an object of lucrative business, the horse has been the focus of attention. Scholars and historians have provided us with much valuable data on the subject. Medieval literature mentions that horse trade brought much wealth in cash to the traders. Many of these traders were from different parts of Kerala and these traders were seen all over South India as donors of generous gifts to temples. At the same time, Wasaf, a Persian historian, visited the western coast some time in the fourteenth century

Translations

A copy of the Hindi translation of the *Sālihōtram* (1381 CE) is found in the royal library at Lucknow. Aufrecht has reported on a medical work of Sālihōtra found in the East India House library.[30] One medical work written by a Salinatha has been found among the Sanskrit manuscripts of Fort William College. The work ascribed to Salinatha is *Rasamatjari*, which deals with the treatments based on different components of mercury. Haji Calfa speaks of an Arabic translation of a Sanskrit veterinary work of Cāṇakya. *Salottar*, a work published in two parts in Calcutta in 1788 and familiar to Arabic and Persian readers is mentioned in the accounts collected by Weber from Berlin Catalogue. This work was composed by a group of scholars and has been translated into Persian by Abdullah Khan who was an emir in the royal

[30] Varier, *History of Āyurveda*, 231.

court of Shah Jahan; it has a translation in English too, by Joseph Ernus. Sir Henry Elliot says that there were two Persian translations by the name *Saluttari*; it is not clear whether Nakula is the author of the original. According to Sir Elliot, the work *Kubrat-ul-mulk* is the Persian translation of *Salottar* rendered during the reign of Feroz Shah Tuglak (1381 CE). This ruler codified the laws and set up many public institutions and translated many Sanskrit works. The Salottar rendered in Persian consists of 11 chapters and 30 sections. Another Persian translation is reported to have been found from Chittore during the conquest of Mevad by Shah Jahan.This is the *Kitab-ul-Vaikkart*; this work, translated by Syed Abdullah Khan Bahadur Feroz Jung, consists of 1,000 verses. Its original work in Sanskrit, it states, is Salottari. There is a translation to *Sālihōtram* in Tibetan too. According to the account of Mitra, the base of the Persian translation of *Sālihōtram* is its Hindi translation by Chetana. Nidhiram Mukherji has compiled a work entitled *Aśvacikitsāsaṅgraha* based on the works of Sālīhotra, Nakula, Bhōjarāja, and Jayadatta.

References to Sālihōtra

Various Purāṇas refer to Aśvāyurveda, Turaṅgaśāstra, and Hastyāyurveda. *Liṅgapurāṇa*, in the context of the discussion on the disciples of Vyāsa, refers to Sālīhotra, Agniveśa, Yuvānasa, and Saradvasu. The fact that Sālīhotra and Agnivesa were classmates points to their date. A work of Sālihōtra is accounted among the manuscript collection of S.R. Bhandarkar, which is a lexical work of Vikramātmaja. But Sālihōtra is nowhere mentioned as a lexicographer. The *Tattvachandrika* quotes Sālihōtra; the author states that both Suśruta and Caraka approve the herb *erandamula* (root of *Ricinus communis*) in the place of *gōkṣura* (*Tribulus terrestris*) in the components of *daśamūla*; Caraka, however, is inclined to *gokṣura*. *Tīkāsarvasva*, a commentary on Amarasimha's *Nāmaliṅgānuśāsanam* (1417–1431) by Sarvānanda, refers to Sālihōtra.

Hastyāyurveda: Treatment for Elephants

According to Hastyāyurveda, Pālakāpya, the author of the voluminous work *Pālakāpyam*, was born to a female elephant who consumed the vital urine of a sage, Sāmagāyana. Some others are of the opinion that

Dhanvantari and Pālakāpya are identical as there is a reference to Suśruta who studied surgery and veterinary science from Dhanvantari. However, there are no other evidences to maintain this contention. Another story tells us that the king Romapada of Campa, a contemporary of Dasaratha, invited Pālakāpya to his country to tame elephants.

Pālakāpyam is an elaborate work on elephants. It deals with elephant diseases and the method of treatment by medicines and scalpels; Burnell terms it as *gajavaidya*. The work is in the form of discussion between the king of Amga and Pālakāpya. It contains the descriptions of the legendary origin of elephants. It also describes general topics concerned with other animals—their types, habits, diseases (106 in number) and remedies, the ways to domesticate them, and so forth. The compilation of this work is after the *Sarasaṅgraha* and appears comparatively to be modern; however, Sarngadhara quotes some verses of Pālakāpya.

Contents of Pālakāpyam

The origin of the knowledge of Hastyāyurveda is traced to Brahma. This work consists of four portions, namely, *Maharogasthāna*, *Kṣudraroga*, *Śalyasthāna*, and *Uttarasthāna*. The first chapter of *Maharogasthāna* narrates the situation that led Pālakāpya to advise Hastyāyurveda to king Romapāda. In addition to this, it describes in great deal a variety of topics, such as the birth of Pālakāpya from a female elephant, the story of how Ruci was cursed by Brahma, the curse of the sage Mātaṅga, the origin of the science, and so forth.

The second chapter deals with the procedures of treatment, such as the application of oil (*abhyaṅga*), bathing (*snana*), and the dietary regimen of elephants. The third chapter describes 15 causes for the death of wild elephants, and their natural food, such as grass and leaves. *Śāstrasaṅgraha*, in its fourth chapter, gives a glimpse of the structure of the text; it elicits that the chapters segregated under four *sthānas*, parts, are in the order of 18, 72, 34, and 36, and there are 20,000 verses in total. The next chapter explains the advantages of keeping elephants and the qualities required for their possessor; the sixth chapter deals with the initiation of disciples. The classification of diseases as inherent, external, *tridoṣika*, curable, incurable, and all serious ailments and their treatments are described in detail in the succeeding chapters. This includes ailments of the eye and eight other types of diseases resulting from the wrong administration of milk, ghee, and intoxicants. There are 72 chapters in the *Kṣudraroga*. They deal elaborately with different types of diseases and the methods of treatment. The next portion, the *Śalyasthāna*, consists of 34 chapters. These chapters discuss symptoms and treatments of various ailments, such as *garbhasambhava*, *garbhavakrānti*, *sarīravichayam śāstragnipraṇidhānam*, *yantravidhi*, *śalyapaharaṇa*, *vidradhi*, and so forth. This portion also deals with the symptoms of rabic poison and its treatment, cuts on vital parts, description of the 15 parts of the body, and so forth. There are 36 chapters in the portion of the *Uttarasthāna*. In these chapters, procedures such as *snehapāna*, *vasti*, *nasya atjana*, and so forth, are discussed. Topics such as dietary regimen, construction of stable for elephants, grass feeding, symptoms of the impending death, shaping of the tusk, methods for improving digestive power and nutrition, use of guggulu (*Commiphora mukul*), milk, garlic preparations, conception, and instructions for attendants, description of urine and castings of cattle, use of salt, and rutting state are dealt with in this portion of the work.

Selected Glossary

ādibalapravṛtta	inherited disease, for example, leprosy, piles
āgantuka	accidental
agni	cautery
agnikṣārakarma	cauterization
āhārya	extraction
amīva	pain
aṉṉapāṉa	food and drink
anūpa	marshy land
ascite	water-belly, probably *mahodara*
Āyurveda	the science of life
bāla	paediatrics
balāsa	swelling
bandhanakarma	bandaging
bhedya	incision
bheṣaja	medicines
bhikṣu	mendicant
bhiṣak	physician
bṛāmhaṇa	building or fattening
chedya	excision
daivabalapravṛtta	superhuman diseases due to witchcraft, cursors
damṣṭra	toxicology
dharma	righteousness (approximately)
doṣa	humour
doṣabalapravṛtta	imbalance in humours due to improper habits, for example, fever
dravyaguṇa	property of herbs and other medicinal objects
dukha	grief

eṣaṇakarma	probing
ēśya	probing
gaṇḍamāla	goitre
graha	demonology or psychiatric treatment
guḍika	a kind of salt
hariman	jaundice
hṛdroga	probably chest pain
jvara	fever
janma balapravṛtta	congenital, for example, deafness, blindness, deformity
jara	geriatrics
jāṅgala	dry zone
kālabalapravṛtta	seasonal, due to seasonal changes
kapha	mucus
karma	action
kāsa	cough
kaṣāya	decoction
kāya	general medicine
kilāsa	leuko-derma
kṛmi	worms
kṣāra	a kind of salt
kuṭa	a kind of salt
langhana	lightening or sliming
lekhanakarma	scraping
madhu	honey
mūla	root
nāḍi	nerve
navanīta	butter
nirdeśa	instructions about treatments
ōṣadhi	medicine
pādapa	generally means tree; etymologically, that which drinks by root
paricāraka	nurse
paśćātkarma	post-operative
pitta	bile
prakṛti	nature
pradhānakarma	principal treat
pūrvakarma	pre-operative
raktamokṣa	blood-letting
rapa	deformity and swelling of limbs

riṣṭalakṣaṇa	signs of death
rūkṣaṇa	roughening
śākha	branch
śalaka	wire, surgical implement used in the treatment of eyes
śalya	surgical tool
samādhi	meditation
sandamśa	bite
saṅgha	Buddhist order
sannipāta	combination
sappi	ghee
śarīra	body
sīvanakriya	suturing
sīvya	suturing
sīvya bandhana	bandaging
sleshma	mucus
snehana	lubricating
śramaṇa	heterodox mendicant
stambhana	arresting
svāsthya	health and moral conduct
svēdana	fomenting
taila	oil
takman	malaria
tridoṣa	three humours
unmāda	insanity
upakalpana	oleation, sudation, emission, and purgation
upayantra	instrument
ūrdhvāṅga	head and the upper limbs
vāta	wind
vedhanakarma	puncturing
vedhya	puncturing
viṣkandha	tetanus
visravaṇakriya	draining
visravia	drainage
vṛṣa	enhancement of sexual potency
yavāgu	gruel
yōjana	formulation

Selected Readings

Sanskrit Original

Carakasamhita. Translated by P.V. Sharma, 6th Edition. Varanasi: Choukhamba Orientalia, 2004.

Suśrutasamhita. Translated by K.R. Srikantha Murthy, 2nd Edition. Varanasi: Choukhamba Orientalia, 2004.

Aṣṭāṅgahṛdaya. Translated by K.R. Srikantha Murthy, 4th Edition. Varanasi: Choukhamba Orientalia. Krishnadas Ayurveda Series, 2004.

Rasavaiśeṣikam. Translated by K. Raghavan Thirumulpad, 4th Edition. Kottakkal: Arya Vaidya Sala, 2018.

Official Publications

Indian Historical Review

Epigraphia Indica (*relevant volumes*)

South Indian Inscriptions, Vol. II, Part III, IV, and V.

———. Vol. III, Part III and IV.

———.Vol. V, Vol. VII, Vol. XXII, and XXIII.

———. *Travancore Archaeological Series*, Vol. III Huzur Office plates.

Books and Journals

Buhler, George. *Indian Paleography*. Calcutta: Indian Studies—Past and Present, 1962.

Chakravarthi, Ranbir, and Krishnendu Ray. 'Healing and Healers Inscribed: Epigraphic Bearing on Healing Houses in Early India'. In *Essays on History of Medicine*, edited by Susmita B. Majumdar and Nayana S. Mukherjee. Mumbai: Indian Institute of Research in Numismatics Studies, 2011.

Cunningham, Alexander. *The Ancient Geography of India*. London: Trubner and Co., 1871.

———. *Corpus Inscriptionum Indicarum*, Vol. 1: Inscriptions of Asoka. Calcutta: Office of the Superintendent of Government Printing, 1877.

Das, Rahul Peter. 'Review of Thite's *Medicine*'. *Indo-Iranian Journal*, 27 (3): 1984, 232–44.

Davids, T.W. Rhys. *Buddhist India*. London: Motilal Banarsidas, 1971 (1903).

Deshpande, Vijaya. 'Indian Influence on Early Chinese Ophthalmology: Glaucoma as a Case Study'. *Bulletin of the School of Oriental and African Studies*, 62 (2): 1999, 306–22.

Dutt, N. *Early Monastic Buddhism*. Calcutta: Firma K.L. Mukhopadhyaya, 1971.

Filliozat, J. *Asokan Inscriptions*. Translated by R.K. Menon. *Indian Studies Past and Present*, Calcutta, 1967.

———. *Classical Doctrines of Indian Medicine*. Delhi: Munshiram Manoharlal, 1964.

Hultzsch, E. *Corpus Inscriptionum Indicarum*, Vol. I: Inscriptions of Asoka. Delhi: Archaeological Survey of India, 1991, reprint.

Jayaswal, K.P. *Hindu Polity: A Constitutional History of India in Hindu Times*, 2nd Edition. Bangalore: Chaukhamba Sanskrit Pratishthan Oriental Publishers & Distributors, 1943.

Kosambi, D.D. *Myth and Reality*. Bombay: Popular Prakashan, 1962.

———. *Culture and Civilization of Ancient India in Historical Outline*. London: Routledge and Kegan Paul, 1965.

———. *Introduction to the Study of Indian History*. Bombay: Popular Prakashan, 1966.

Krishnaswamy N. *Āyurveda*. Chennai: Vidyaprakash Publication, 2013.

Kumar, Deepak. *Science and the Raj 1857–1905*. Delhi: Oxford India Paperbacks, 1997.

Madihassan, S. 'Comparative Study of the Early Systems of Indian Cosmology and the Tridosha Humeral Doctrine'. *Indian Journal of History and Science*, 15 (2): 1980, 223–9.

Majumdar, Susmita Basu, and Nayana Sharma Mukherjee. *Essays on History of Medicine*. Mumbai: IIRNS, 2013.

Motichandra. *Sarthavahan*, translated by K.N. Ezhuthachan. Delhi: Kerala Sahitya Akademi, 1956.

Mukharjee, R.K. *Asoka*. Calcutta: Vivekananda International Foundation, Calcutta, 1928.

Needham, Joseph. *Science and Civilization in China*. Cambridge: Needham Research Institute, 1954–2004.

Olivelle, Patrick, Janice Leoshko, and Himanshu Prabha Ray, eds. *Reimagining Asoka: Memory and History*. Delhi: Oxford University Press, 2012.

Pischel, R. *Comparative Grammar of the Prakrit Language*. Translated by Subhadra Jha, 2nd Edition. Delhi, Motilal Banarsidas, 1965.

Prasad, Jwala. *History of Indian Epistemology*, 3rd Edition. Delhi: Munshiram Manoharlal, 1987.

Prinsep, James. *Essays on Indian Antiquities, Historic, Numismatic, and Palaeographic, of the Late James Prinsep*. Vols I and II. London: John Murray, 1858.

Raghava Varier, M.R. *Rediscovery of Ayurveda*. Delhi: Viking, and Kottakkal: Aryavaidyasala, 2005.

Raghava Varier, M.R. and Nhayath Balan Srikrishnan, ed. *Alathur Maṇipravāḷam*, text with commentary. Kottakkal: Arya Vaidya Sala, 2009.

Ray, Himanshu P. *Monastery and Guild*. Delhi: Oxford University Press, 1986.

Sastri, A. M. *Outline of Early Buddhism*. Varanasi: Indological Book House, 1965.

Sewell, Robert. *A Forgotten Empire*, new edition. Delhi: Cultural Publication Department, 1996.

Sharma, P.V. *Caraka Samhita*, Jai Krishna Ayurveda Series. Varanasi and Delhi: Chaukhamba Orientalia, 1981.

Sharma, R.S. *Material Culture and Social Formations in Ancient India*. Delhi: Macmillan India, 1983 (1969).

Smith, V.A. *Asoka: The Buddhist Emperor of India*, 3rd Edition. Oxford: Clarendon Press, 1920.

Srikantha Murthy, K.R. *Susruta Samhita*, 2nd edition. Varanasi/Delhi: Choukhambha Orientalia, 2004.

Thapar, Romila. *Asoka and the Decline of Mauryas*. Oxford: Oxford University Press, 1961.

———. *Ancient Indian Social History*. Delhi: Oxford University Press, 1984.

Thite, G.U. *Medicine in Its Magico-religious Aspects According to the Vedic and Later Literature*. Poona: Continental Prakashan, 1982.

Valiathan, M.S. *Legacy of Caraka*. Hyderabad: Universities Press Pvt. Ltd, 2007.

———. *Legacy of Suśruta*. Hyderabad: Universities Press Pvt. Ltd, 2007.

———. *Legacy of Vāgbhaṭa*. Hyderabad: Universities Press Pvt. Ltd, 2007.

———. *An Introduction to Ayurveda*. Hyderabad: Universities Press Pvt. Ltd, 2013.

Varier, N.V.K. *History of Āyurveda*. 56, Kottakal Ayurveda Series. Kottakkal: Arya Vaidya Sala, 2012.

Zysk, Kenneth G. *Medicine in the Veda*. Delhi: Motilal Banarsidass Publishers Pvt. Ltd, 1998.

Index

ācārarasāyana, 54
ācāryas (perceptors), 14, 40–1, 44, 55, 61, 64, 66, 77–8, 134; advise to students, 49; lineage of, 43; of medicine, 96; qualities of, 48; of surgical treatments, 83
Acharya, Yadavji Trikramji, 120
ādibalapravṛtta (inherited disease), 75
agada tantra (toxicology), 8–9, 20–1, 78–9
agnikarma (cauterization), 74; materials used for, 74–5; types of, 75
Agniveśa, 41, 44–5, 63, 87–9, 96
Agniveśatantra, xxvi, 44, 63
Aithareya Brāhmaṇa, 9, 20, 123
ākāśa (ether), 6, 76, 90, 143, 145
Ālattūr Maṇipravāḷam, 113
alchemy: in *Atharvaveda*, 131; characteristics of, 130; concept of, 130; mantras and, 134–5; medicines and elixirs, 130–2; mental and physical accomplishments, 133; Nāgārjuna, 133–4; philosophy of mercury, 135–6; physiological, 134; processes essential to, 135; *rasa* therapy, 130
amputation, xxx; and grafting, 4–5, 75
anatomic dissection: instruments used for, 67; knowledge of, 49–50; manual for, 28; mode of, 67; in *Suśrutasamhita*, 27; in thirteenth and fourteenth centuries, 28
anatomy, knowledge of, xxiv, 10–11, 27–8; monastic knowledge, 26–9
animal anatomy, knowledge of: in Greek culture, 28; in Western countries, 27–8
animals: physiology of, 150; treatment of: *See* veterinary science
animal urine: as Āyurvedic medicine, 32; for treatment for snake bites, 32
Annals of the Royal Botanic Gardens, 145
aphrodisiacs, use of, 92
Arthaśāstra, 134, 137–8
Ashoka, Emperor: and Buddhist *saṅghas*, 102; Rock Edict II of, 101, 136
Asiatic Society of Bengal, xvi
Aṣṭāṅga Ayurveda, 92, 97

Aṣṭāṅgahṛdaya, xxvii, 42, 77, 87, 89–90, 91–4, 100, 109; *Āyurvedarasāyana* of, 111; *Cikitsasthāna*, 93; Great Triad (*Bṛhtrayi*) of Āyurveda, 92; historical importance of, 91; *Kalpasthāna*, 94; nature and contents of, 92–4; *Nidānasthāna*, 93; *Śārīrasthāna*, 93; *Sarvāṅgasundari*, 91; on social customs and practices, 92; *Sūtrasthāna*, 93; *Uttarasthāna*, 94
Aṣṭāṅgasaṅgraha, xxvii, 89–90, 91–2
Aṣṭavaidyans of Kerala, 113
Aśvaghōṣa, 154–5
Aśvāyurveda (treatment of horses), xxiii, 42, 146, 147–9; Boghazkeui inscription of, 146; on physiology of animals, 150
Aśvinidevas, 4, 9, 131
Atharvaveda, xxvii, xxiv–xxv, 4, 5, 8–11, 13–14, 41, 102, 127, 137; ideas about alchemy, 131
Ātreya, Punarvasu, 29, 42, 55, 62, 63, 89, 96, 137
āturaśālais (health centres), xxvii, 58, 106, 108, 109, 127–8; Vīracōḻan *āturaśālai*, 106
auṣadhi, 139
Āyurveda: approaches for treatment of diseases in, 76–7; *Aṣṭāṅga* Āyurveda, 92, 97; beyond the Indian subcontinent, 99–100; Brahma's, 42–3; branches of, 79; and Buddhist monastic medicine, 30; Caraka views on, 59; Chinese translations of, 99; empirico-rational medicine of, 100; geographical base of, xxi; history of, xviii; knowledge of, xxiii, xxviii, 40; principles of, 59; setback under British occupation, 118; in Tibetan Buddhism, 100; Vedic origin of, xxiv, 40
bālacikitsa (paediatrics), 92, 94, 115
Benaras Hindu University (BHU), 119
Bengal Asiatic Society, 145
Bhattāraka, Savarṇan Aśvatthāmā, 106
Bheḷa, 29, 40, 96; study of the mind, 88
Bhēḷasamhita, 87, 88
bheṣaja, *See* Vedic medicine
bhikṣus (medicant saints), xxiv, 25, 33, 44, 125
bhiṣak (the healer), 12, 17–18, 21, 95–6; medicinal knowledge of, 124
Bimbisāra (king of Magadha), 25, 34
Bishagacharya, G.N. Mukhopadhyaya, xix
black magic, 11
bōdhisattva, 96
Bodhisatva Bhaiṣajyarājan, 99
Bower manuscript, xix, 29, 99, 153
Brāhmaṇas, 5–6, 10, 23, 40; in later Vedic literature, 9–10; *Śatapatha Brāhmaṇa*, 9
Bṛhadsamhita, 38, 138, 140, 143
British Raj, xvi, 117–18, 128
Buddhist monastic tradition of medicine, 24, 30, 96; yogic practices, 30–2
Buddhist Monastic universities, 97
Buddhist *saṅghas*, 25, 63, 127; development of the materia medica in, 32–3; medical care to the *bhikṣus*, 96, 125; programmes of compassion, 99
Buddhist *vihāras* (monasteries), xxiii, 102, 127

Calcutta Madrasa, 118
Calcutta Medical College, 119
Calcutta Sanskrit School, 118
Caraka, xxvi, 14, 29, 33, 42, 44–5, 87–8; concept of yoga, 62–3;

contributions of, 63–5; epistemology of, 61–3; version of Samhitas, 41; views on Āyurveda, 59
Carakasamhita, xxvi–xviii, xix–xxi, 7, 29, 45–7, 67, 97, 109, 121; Āragvadhīya, 131; *Cikitsasthāna* in, 47, 78, 93, 131, 151, 152; on classes of physicians, 54–5; codification of, 63; commentary by Gangadhara Ray on, 118–19; on medical education, 97–8; on modalities of medical treatment, 51–2; on nursing homes, 58; *pañcakarma*, 52–3; on procedure of medical treatment, 50–1; *rasāyana* therapy, 59–61; *Śārīrasthāna* of, 46, 63–4; on diagnosis of diseases, 64; *vājīkaraṇa* therapy, 59–61; *Vimānasthāna* of, 46, 131
cataract surgery, xxii, xxix, 126; knowledge of, 79–80, 126
celestial physicians, 4, 9, 13
Chakraborthy, Haranachandra, 118–19
Chatopadhyaya, Deviprasad, 18, 56
chemistry, origin of, 130–1
cikitsa (treatment), process of, 67, 76–7, 97, 127
cikitsāsthāna, 45, 47, 67, 78
classification of foods in, 33

daily routine (*dinacarya*), observance of, 54, 57, 65
daivavyapāśraya (magico-religious) tradition, xviii
Ḍalhaṇa, 33
damṣtra (toxicology), 92, 94
dehaṇmānasa (psychosomatic principle), 64
Dhanvantari, 41, 42, 43, 66, 151, 153, 157
Dhanvantari, 120, 122
Dharmaśāstras, xvi, 4, 25, 26, 96, 98, 104, 126, 150
dhātus (constituent elements of the body), 59, 61
diseases: causation of, 23–6; empirico-rational idea of, 20; magico-religious and ritual treatment of, 20; management of, 32–4; *siroroga* (diseases of the head), 94; skin diseases, 131; treating of, 76–7; types of, 75–6
disinfection of wounds, 74
dissection of the body *See* anatomic dissection
Divodāsa (Dhanvantari), 41–2, 66–7
doṣa (bodily humour), xxiv, 46, 52, 75
dravyaguṇa (property of herbs and other medicinal objects), 40, 89
Dṛḍhabala, 45, 47, 131
drugs: classification of, 84; rules pertaining to, 24

East India Company: administrative policy of, xviii; surgeons of, xvii
Ègveda hymns, 4, 11, 131
elixir, synthesis of, 130–2
empirico-rational medicine, 100, 102, 104, 127
Enlightened One, 22, 29, 66, 125

Fâ-hien, 58
Firdaus Al-Hikma, 90
flesh, grafting of, 75
fumigation, 74

gaṇḍūṣavidhi (methods of oral cleaning), 78
Ganga–Yamuna doab, 7, 24, 127, 147; human settlements in, 138
Gautama Buddha, 22–3, 29, 31, 33, 66, 125

Goma Maṭha, Tibet, 133
grahacikitsa (treatment of illness caused by attack of demons), 86, 92, 94
Greek medical traditions, xviii–xix, xx, xxi, 28, 84
guggulu (*Commiphora mukul*), 15, 56, 74, 158
Guṇaratna, 142–3
gurukula (teacher's residence) system, 53, 97, 115, 118

Harappan culture *See* Indus Valley civilization
Hārīta, 40, 89, 96
Hārītasamhita, 89, 153
Harṣacarita, 132–3
Hastyāyurveda (treatment for elephants), 42, 156–7, 158
health routine (*svasthavṛtta*), observance of, 54
herbal medicine, 2, 15
herbal plants: importance of, 136; worship of, 2, 12, 136
hospital (*ārōgya vihara* or *ārōgyaśāla*), 38, 111
Hsuan-tsang (Chinese pilgrim), 58, 96–7, 133
human anatomy, 10–11, 26–7, 28–9; codification of, 28

impending death (*riṣṭas*), symptoms of, 76
Indian Science Congress, 145
indigenous knowledge of healing and healthcare, 8, 40; British policy towards, 118; in Harappan culture, 123; origin and development of, 123
indigenous medicine, knowledge of, 112
Indra, Lord, 13, 17, 40–1, 44, 104
Indus Valley civilization, 88; development and diseases, 7–8; early history on art of healing, 8–9; Eastward migration of the Vedic people, 5–6; end of, 3; healing and healthcare system in, 1–2, 123; herbal medicines, 2; historical developments of, 6–7; inter-tribal conflicts, 5; later Vedic literature, 9–10; mutual conflicts and warfare, 7; rise and growth of urban settlements, 6–7; surgical operations in, 3; Vedic society, 4–5; worship of herbal plants, 2, 136
Itihāsa–Purāṇa tradition, 142
I-Tsing (Chinese pilgrim), 97

Janapadas (human settlement), 7–8
janmabalapravṛtta (congenital disease), 75
jarācikitsa, 92, 94
Jīvaka Pustakam, 29
Jīvaka, story of, 17, 54, 66, 86, 96, 137; in Jaina Works, 35–6; in *Kāśyapasamhita*, 34–5, 41; as K'i-yu in Chinese language, 99; in *Mahāvagga*, 33–4
Jvarasamuccaya, 85

kālabalapravṛtta (seasonal disease), 75
Kaḷari system, formation of, 114
kālavāda, 62, 77
Kalpasthāna, 45, 47, 78, 86, 131
Kaniṣka, King, 45, 154–5
karmayogya, 50
Kāśyapasamhita, 34–5, 41, 53, 56, 78, 85–7; Chinese translation of, 99
Kauḷa system, of the Śaiva cult, 133
kaumārabhṛtya (paediatrics), 33, 35, 85, 126
Kautalya's *Arthaśāstra*, 8, 26, 81, 134, 140, 150
kāyacikitsa (general medicine), 40, 46, 80, 90, 92–3

Komārabhacca, Jīvaka *See* Jīvaka, story of
Kṛtayuga (the Golden Age), 41, 43
Kubrat-ul-mulk (Persian translation of *Salottar*), 156

labour room (*sūtikāgāra*), 58
leeches, use of, 74–5
Legacy of Suśruta, The, xxvii
leprosy, treatment of, 131

magico-religious healing, Vedic perfomance of, 124
Mahābhārata: Śāntiparva of, 62, 143
mahābhūtas, principles of, 78
Mahāvagga, 29, 31–3; story of Jīvaka, 33; story of Kāśyapa, 35
Mahāyāna Buddhism, 45, 99–100, 132
Majumdar, Susmita Basu, xxix–xxx
Manusmṛti, 81, 126, 150
marma vidya, 114, 116
maṭha (residence of Brahmins), 109, 111
Mauryan period, medicinal services in, 36–9, 38; Buddhist monasteries and, 36; Girnar Edict II of Ashoka, 36–7
medical education (*cikitsa vidya*), 10, 97, 98; in ancient India, 96; in Buddhist monastic institutions, 29, 96; at Calcutta Madrasa, 118; at Calcutta Sanskrit School, 118; earliest form of, 95–6; *gurukula* (teacher's residence) system, 97; institutionalization of, 96; Nālanda University, 97; selection of a medical student, 97; Takṣasila (Taxila) university, 96
medical ethics, development of, 24, 125
medical institutions, 109–12; remuneration given to staff members of, 110
medical knowledge: acquisition of, 29, 96; among ascetic wanderers, 31; developments in medieval Kerala, 112–16; of indigenous medicine, 112; in Jainism, 31; traced to Hindu divinities, 104; transmission of, 47
medical services, in Hindu religious centres, 104
medical treatment: modalities of, 51–2; procedure of, 50–1
medicinal doctrines in India, xix
medicinal herbs, 8; instinctive use of, 13; knowledge of, 65; *oṣadhi*, 12; qualities of, 13; worship of, 136
medicine, 29–30, 49; animal urine as, 32; Buddhist idea of, 26, 30–1; connection with Chinese treatment, 99; elixirs, 130–2; history of, 9; Jaina tradition of, 31; in Mauryan period, 36–9; military medicine, 83; monastery and, 30–2; Sikh monks tradition of, 30; use of food as, 31; Vedic medicine, 11–12
mercury, philosophy of, 131, 134, 135–6
military medicine, 83
Mitra (Vedic god), 10, 20
mokṣa (eternal liberation from birth and death), 54; attaining, 62, 63
Mukherjee, Nayana Sharma, xxix–xxx

Nāgārjuna, 29, 133–4; compendia of medicine, 31
Nālanda *mahāvihāra*, 96–7
nāsācikitsa (rhinology), 94
netracikitsa (ophthalmology), 94, 115
Nidānasthāna, 46, 47, 77
Nikāyas, xxiv–xxv, 23, 33
nursing homes, 58

oṣadhi (medicinal herbs), 12, 15, 131
osteology, knowledge of, 11

Pālakāpyam, 156; contents of, 157–8
Paḷḷibhagavathi Temple, Palakkad, 104
pancabhūta (five basic elements), xxiv, xxvii, 46, 61, 63, 76, 90
pañcakarma programme, 52–3, 60
parīkṣa (investigation and diagnosis of diseases), 64
peccant humours, concept of, 26
physicians: classes of, 54–5; status of, 17–19
Piṭakas, xxiv–xxv, 23, 33
plant diseases, 139–40, 141–3, 144–5; in medieval period, 143–4; in modern period, 144–5
plants: classification of, 138; herbal plants, 2, 12, 136; worship of, 2, 12, 136
plastic surgery, xviii, 83
poisons: of animal origin (*jaṅgamaviṣa*), 78–9; of plant origin (*sthāvaraviṣa*), 78–9; use of, 8
Prajāpati, 42, 86
prakṛti (basic nature): of human body, xxvii, 61–2
prāṇābhisara, 49, 54
prasūtiśāla (maternity house), 111
Pratyakṣaśārīra, 88, 119
Purāṇas: *Agnipurāṇa*, 42; *Brahmavaivarta purāṇa*, 42
purgative drugs, 76, 94, 139

raktamokṣa (blood-letting), 52, 53, 67, 83, 89
rapas, 12
rasāyana (rejuvenation) therapy, 7, 47, 54, 58, 59–61, 67, 78, 130; *kuṭīprāveśika*, 60; modes of, 60; parts of, 59–60; *rasa*, 59
Ravigupta's *Siddhasāra*, 29
Ray, Gangadhara, 118–19
Report on Vernacular Education, 118
Rgveda, xxiv–xxv, 5, 102, 131, 146; on healing and healthcare, 8; *maṇḍalas* of, 9, 12, 15–17, 136; on medicinal herbs, 8
rhinoplasty, treatment of, 26, 80–1
riṣṭalakṣaṅa (signs of ailment), 40, 89
Rock Edict II of Ashoka, xxi, 101, 136
Roy, Yaminibhushan, 119

sadhya (competent nurses), qualities of, 33
sadvṛtta (code of conduct for ideal life), 54, 78
sadyovraṇas (sudden injuries), 78
Sage Bharadvāja, 41
Sage Kāśyapa, 86; on paediatrics, 42; story of, 35, 40; version of Samhitas, 41–2
Sage Mātaṅga, 42
Sage Pāṇini, 151
Sage Patañjali, 62; *Aṣṭādhyāyi*, 66; concept of yoga, 62–3
Sage Sālīhōtra, 42, 151–3; *Aśvalakṣaṇaśāstra*, 154; *Aśvapraśamsa*, 154; medical work of, 155; nativity of, 151; references to, 156; *Sālihōtram*, 151–3
Sage Surapāla, 42
Sage Vāgbhaṭa, xxvii, 42, 60, 87, 89–91, 109, 113
Sage Vasishta, 86
śālākyatantra, 81, 119, 126
Sālātureeya, 151
Sālihōtram, 151; contents of, 151–3; Hindi translation of, 155; Suśruta in, 153; Tibetian translation of, 156
Salottar, 155; Persian translation of, 156
śalyacikitsa (surgery), 8, 92, 94

Samhitas, *ācāryas* of, 40–1; on ancient Indian system of medicine, 40; in *Aṣṭāṅgahṛdaya*, 42; *Bhēḷasamhita*, 87; Caraka's version of, 41, 44–5, 46–7, 63–5; dissection of the body, 49–50; *Hārītasamhita*, 89; initiation of the disciple, 48–9; Kāśyapa's version of, 41–2, 85–7; legend in the Purāṇas, 42–4; procedure of treatment, 50–1; Suśruta's version of, 41
saṅghata balapravṛtta (incidental disease), 76
Sānkhya school of philosophy, 124
Śārīrasthāna, 46, 62, 63
Śārṅgadhara, 143, 154
Śastracikitsa, 92
Śatapatha Brāhmaṇa, 5, 9, 11, 21, 123
Sātavāhanas, 39, 134
Sen, Ganganatha, 118–19
Sen, Yogendranath, 118
Sharma, P.V., xxi, 63, 121
siddhas (holy men), of Śaiva system, 132–3
Siddhisthāna, 45, 47, 131, 152
Śīlāditya II, King, 58
Skandapurāṇa, 58
skin diseases, 131
Socrates, xvi
Soma, 9, 131
śramaṇas (Buddhist monks), 23, 31
Surgical Ethics in Āyurveda, 121
surgical instruments, 68, 69–72
surgical operations: administration of ghee, 74–5; code of conduct of physicians, 74; disinfection of wounds, 74; fumigation, process of, 74; grafting of flesh, 75; of the head, 34; in Indus Civilization, 3; *paścātkarma* (post-operative treatment), 68; phases of, 68; for piles and calculus, 78; *pūrvakarma* (pre-operative treatment), 68; for removal of cataract, 79–80; rhinoplasty, 26, 80–1; role of climate in, 74; tools and instruments used for, 68, 69–72; training in, 81–2, 83–4; use of leeches in, 74–5
Suśruta, xvi, xxvi, 14, 29, 33, 42, 54, 66–7, 86, 88, 131, 140; on poison, 78; on ideal age for sexual union, 78; on interdisciplinary learning, 80; on paediatrics, 78; on treatment, 59; surgical tools designed by, 68
Suśrutasamhita, xxvi, 8, 26, 40, 45, 53, 67, 83, 119, 121, 126; *agada tantra* (toxicology), 8; Chakraborthy's commentary on, 119; descriptions of food and drink in, 77; on ill-effects of polluted medicines and diet, 74; knowledge of the human body, 27; on phases of surgery, 68; on rhinoplasty, 80–1; *Sūtrasthāna*, 46, 62, 67–8; on training in surgery, 81–3, 84; *Uttaratantra*, 79–80; *See also* surgical operations
Sūtrasthāna, 46, 62, 67–8, 77
svēdana (fomenting/sweating), 51, 58, 78; sweat room (*svedagṛha*), 58

takman (malaria), 9, 16, 19
Takṣasila (Taxila) university, 29, 96
Thapar, Romila, 22, 30, 43–4
tools and instruments, used for surgery, 68, 69–72; designed by Suśruta, 68; metallurgical skills in making, 73; proliferation of, 73; types of, 69–72
treatment of diseases, in Āyurvedic system, 61; *bālacikitsa*, 92, 94;

grahacikitsa, 86, 92, 94; *kāyacikitsa*, 80; *rasāyana* therapy, *See rasāyana* (rejuvenation) therapy; *śalyacikitsa*, 8, 92, 94; *śamana cikitsa*, 77; *śodhana cikitsa*, 76–7; *vājīkaraṇa* (aphrodisiacs) therapy, 59–61; *yuktivyapāśraya* (empirico-rational) therapy, 63
tridoṣa, theory of, 23, 63, 74, 76, 125, 136

Uttaratantra, 53, 67, 79–80, 126
Ūrdhvāṅgacikitsa, 92

Vaiśeṣika guṇas, xxvi, 62
Vaiśeṣika School of philosophy, 21, 62, 64, 91, 124
vājīkaraṇa (aphrodisiacs) therapy, 7, 47, 59–61, 67
Valiathan, M.S., xxv–xxvii, xxviii
vamana (vomiting), 47, 52, 53, 58, 76, 78
Varier, N.V.K., 86
Varier, P.S., 119, 122
vasti (enema), 50, 52, 53, 89
Vedic healing: epistemology of, 19; nature and content of, 12–17; nomenclature of ailments in, 16
Vedic medicine, 11–12; *oṣadhi* (medicinal herbs), 12; practitioners of, 19; prescription of regular medicines, 14; preservation and transmission of knowledge, 19–21
Vedic society: art of healing in, 8–9; cattle wealth, 5; eastward migration of people, 5–6; inter-tribal conflicts, 5; social differentiation in, 17; status of physicians in, 17–19
Velans community, 101–2, 113; healing practices of, 102
veterinary science, 146–8, 149–50; accomplishments in, 149; Aśvāyurveda, 146, 147–9; Hastyāyurveda, 42, 156–7; and horticulture in ancient India, 149–50
Vīrarājēndra, King, 106
virecana (purgation), 47, 52, 78
Vṛkṣāyurveda (treatment of trees and plants), xxiii, 42, 136–7, 138–9; classification of plants, 138; on plant diseases, 139–41, 142–5

Wan Hsuan Tse (Chinese pilgrim), 135

yajña (Vedic ritual), 5–6, 10, 21, 56
yoga, concept of, 62–3, 88

Zysk, Kenneth G., xxiii–xxiv, xxiv–xxv, 17, 97, 103

About the Author

M.R. Raghava Varier is director general at the Centre for Heritage Studies, Department of Culture, Government of Kerala, at Thrippunithura, Kerala. Prior to this, he was a consultant at the Museum of Ayurveda, Arya Vaidya Sala, Kottakal, Kerala, and chief editor at their Department of Publication before that. He was also visiting professor at the Department of History, Malayalam University, Tirur, Kerala, and M.G. University, Kottayam, Kerala, among others.

He received his training in epigraphy under the Directorate of Epigraphy, Mysore, Karnataka. He completed his PhD at Calicut University, Kerala; M.Phil at Jawaharlal Nehru University (JNU), Delhi; and M.A. at Calicut University. His recent publications include the Kerala Archaeological Series (2010), published under the Government of Kerala, as well as books such as *Aspects of Jainism in Kerala* (forthcoming), *Studies in South Indian Palaeography* (forthcoming), and *A History of Kerala* (2018, with Rajan Gurukkal).